When Someone You Love Needs Nursing Home, Assisted Living, or In-Home Care

The Complete Guide

Second Edition

WHEN SOMEONE YOU LOVE NEEDS NURSING HOME, ASSISTED LIVING, OR IN-HOME CARE

The Complete Guide

SECOND EDITION

ROBERT F. BORNSTEIN, PH.D.
AND
MARY A. LANGUIRAND, PH.D.

NEWMARKET PRESS · NEW YORK

Second edition 2009

This book is published in the United States of America and in Canada.

10   9   8   7   6   5   4   3   2   1

ISBN 978-1-55704-822-6 (Hardcover edition)
ISBN 978-1-55704-816-5 (Paperback edition)

Library of Congress Cataloging-in-Publication Data

Bornstein, Robert F.
When someone you love needs nursing home, assisted living, or in-home care
: the complete guide / Robert F. Bornstein And Mary A. Languirand. — 2nd ed.
p. cm.
Rev. ed. of: When someone you love needs nursing home care. 1st ed. c2001.
Includes bibliographical references and index.
ISBN 978-1-55704-822-6 (hardcover : alk. paper) — ISBN 978-1-55704-816-5
(pbk. : alk. paper) 1. Nursing homes. 2. Nursing home care. 3. Consumer education. I. Languirand, Mary A. II. Bornstein, Robert F. When someone you love
needs nursing home care. III. Title.
RA997.B67 2009
362.16—dc22   2008054291

QUANTITY PURCHASES
Companies, professional groups, clubs, and other organizations may qualify
for special terms when ordering quantities of this title. For information, write
to Special Sales Department, Newmarket Press, 18 East 48th Street,
New York, NY 10017; call (212) 832-3575; fax (212) 832-3629 or
e-mail mailbox@newmarketpress.com.

www.newmarketpress.com

Designed by M.J. DiMassi

Manufactured in the United States of America

To Our Parents

Diane and Lewis Bornstein

Helen and Alfred Languirand

Contents

3. *In-Home Care: Autonomy, Continuity, and a Bit of Extra Help* 30

4. *When In-Home Care Becomes Impossible: Screaming, Crying, Fighting...and Moving On* 48

11. 🖎 *When Things Get Better:*
The Transition Back Home 191

12. 🖎 *When It's Time to Let Go: Hospice and Beyond* 211

✤ *Checklists, Worksheets, and Resources* *235*

Preface

We wrote this book for you: the person whose loved one needs some extra help and care. Whether your loved one is a parent, spouse, or sibling, please know you're not alone. There are more than forty million caregivers in America—people just like you, who want to help but don't have experience dealing with Alzheimer's disease, stroke, and other late-life health problems.

This book will help you navigate the complex, intimidating bureaucracy of today's eldercare system. We provide bottom-line, no-nonsense, practical information to help your loved one get the best care possible during every stage of the process, from the earliest signs of illness, through in-home care and assisted living, to the nursing home, and beyond. We discuss late-life medical problems and their treatments, of course, but we don't stop there. We also discuss the psychological, legal, and financial aspects of in-home and out-of-home care, so you can help your loved one anticipate all the different issues that arise before, during, and after treatment. By the time you finish this book, you'll understand our time-tested, practical framework for caregiving, plus strategies for dealing with every aspect of in-home and out-of-home care.

Because caregiving begins with you, the caregiver, our framework for caregiving includes plenty of advice designed to help you cope during this challenging process. Your loved one needs your help and support, but remember: Good caregiving means taking good care of yourself as well. We'll show you how.

We believe you'll benefit most from this book if you begin with those sections that are most relevant to your loved one's current situation. For many caregivers, that means starting with Chapter 1. If your loved one's health has already declined somewhat, you should begin with those chapters that discuss what he or she needs right now. You can always go back and read the other chapters later (and we recommend that you do, because these chapters contain information that will be useful to you down the line).

Throughout this book, we provide contact information you can use to learn more about specific issues (for example, Medicare, elder law, caregiver stress). We provide telephone and Internet contact information whenever these are available, but make no mistake: In most cases you'll find it easier to access needed information over the Internet than by phone. Among other things, the Internet is open twenty-four hours a day (even on weekends), and it never puts you on hold (well, almost never). If you don't have Internet access, consider getting it. If you can't afford it, contact local libraries, colleges, and universities. They often provide free Internet access for members of the community.

A word about language: We don't mince words. So when we refer to "dementia," or a "demented nursing home resident," we're not trying to be unkind or make light of the situation. "Dementia" is the accepted medical term for the confusion and memory impairment that result from Alzheimer's disease and other medical conditions. We're using such terms so you'll be familiar with them when you discuss your loved one's care with physicians, insurers, and others.

A warning: It's impossible to discuss late-life health care without mentioning things like fecal incontinence, urinary tract infections, and other topics that are not (shall we say) typical dinner table conversation. As we note in Chapter 9, "old age ain't for sissies," but we believe it's best to discuss these things in a straightforward manner, rather than hiding behind more palatable (but less accurate) terms.

We'd like to thank a number of people who contributed greatly to this book, and without whom we could not have written it. First and foremost, we'd like to thank Esther Margolis, president of Newmarket Press, who recognized the value of our approach and signed the project. When the first edition of the book had such a positive impact on many people's lives, it was

Esther who encouraged us to write a revised and updated edition.

Several other members of the Newmarket Press team made key contributions to this project and taught us a great deal along the way. We'd like to thank Jim Ellison, Keith Hollaman, Michelle Howry, and Linda Carbone for their editorial expertise, patience, and skill; together they helped shape our words into sparkling text. Harry Burton and Meredith Hirsch did a tremendous job promoting our book, ensuring that it would reach the broadest possible audience. We are grateful to Mary Jane DiMassi, whose innovative design gave *When Someone You Love Needs Nursing Home, Assisted Living, or In-Home Care* a compelling appearance that complemented and supported our message; her efforts helped pull the entire package together.

Finally, we'd like to thank our agent, Joelle Delbourgo, whose support and enthusiasm helped transform our ideas into something tangible—the book you're now holding in your hands. Without her energy, patience, skill, and encouragement, this book would never have been written.

1

The Invisible Army

Driving home from work, Patricia felt terrific. Business was picking up, and after two tough years, she was finally turning a profit. The kids were healthy, Jim was well, and the holidays were just around the corner. By this time next week the house would be full of people—Mom, Elizabeth, Jim's parents and brother, Andrew back from college for his first visit home. Patricia smiled to herself, turned up the radio. All her hard work, all her planning, was finally paying off.

When Patricia pulled into the driveway, she knew right away that something was wrong. She could see Elizabeth's face in the window, and as the headlights flashed across the house, her daughter turned away. When Patricia reached the door, it was already open. Elizabeth stood there, eyes wide with fright.

"Mom, Nana's sick. The hospital just called."

Patricia felt a chill run down her back. "When?" she asked. Her voice was barely a whisper.

"Just now. Just a minute ago. Right before you got here."

Patricia felt dizzy. She took a deep breath. She stood still for a moment, trying to comprehend. Her mother, sick? How? What happened?

Twenty minutes later, she arrived at the hospital. It was chaos: phones ringing, people rushing everywhere, a loudspeaker squawking, an automatic door shushing open and shut. Patricia made her way to the desk and explained why she was there. The nurse looked puzzled for a moment, then she seemed to relax. When she spoke her voice was soft, reassuring.

Her mother, the nurse explained, had fallen in the bathtub and broken her hip. They were taking X rays now, and then they would set it. After that Patricia could go up and see her. It might take a while, so maybe Patricia should get a cup of coffee or something to eat. They'd call her when her mother was ready.

Patricia sat and waited, paced and fretted, then sat and waited some more. Hours passed. Finally, they called her in....

By the time Patricia got home, it was past midnight. She was scared and tired and very confused, with a million questions and no good answers. Was Mom going to be OK? What did they mean, "hook up with Social Services"? What's a rehab center, anyway, and how do I find one? How am I going to pay for all this? What if I can't pay for it? Will I lose the business? The house?

Patricia sat in her car and sobbed. All my planning, she thought, all my hard work, and now it's gone, it's all falling apart. What do I do now? Where do I go from here?

It took Patricia a few minutes to pull herself together. She stayed in the car until her tears had dried and her breathing had returned to normal. Then she went inside. She and Jim had a lot of talking to do.

Does this sound familiar? If your experience is anything like Patricia's, then like her, you've been drafted into an "invisible army," now forty million strong and growing. Members of this army aren't soldiers; they're caregivers. They come from all walks of life—young and old, rich and poor, married, single, widowed, and divorced, and from every religious and ethnic background. Members of this army are all very different, but they have one thing in common: a loved one who may soon need in-home, assisted living, or nursing home care.

What brought you to this invisible army of caregivers? Was it a frail and aging parent who fell in the tub? A confused spouse who can no longer remember to turn off the stove—no matter how many times you remind her? A sibling, perhaps, who can't drive anymore, and with no one to turn to but you?

We don't have to tell you this is not an easy time to be a caregiver. Years ago, your job would have been easier. For one thing, people didn't live nearly as long as they do today, and far fewer people spent time in a skilled nursing facility. Ailing family members were cared for at home back then, and relatives tended to live close to one another, enabling everyone to share caregiving duties more easily. The number of out-of-home care options was far more limited.

Shifting economic and demographic trends have made caregiving more complex than ever before. Financial pressures now require most adults to work outside the home. Typical two-parent households are no longer the norm, and single parents have less time and fewer resources to devote to their parents or aging siblings. Career demands often require people to live far from their roots. Even those of us who come from cultures that have traditionally taken great pride in caring for elders at home may find that the demands of modern living make this nearly impossible.

Advances in medicine have also made things more complicated for caregivers, because seriously ill family members often live for many years. Medicine has been a blessing, but it creates some new responsibilities as well—responsibilities that fall upon people like you, the son or daughter, wife or husband, sister or brother, nephew or niece, who wants only the best for the person you love.

Welcome to the invisible army.

Eldercare Myths and Misperceptions

We know a woman who put a caveat in her will. The caveat stated that if either of her sons ever placed her in a nursing home, that son would inherit nothing.

This woman's fear is understandable, of course: Who among us wants to spend time in a nursing home? But what a mistake she made! She might as well have put a line in her will that said, "I expressly forbid my sons from getting me the best care possible if I ever become seriously ill."

It sounds silly when you say it that way, so why would our friend have done this? Probably because she has a vivid, frightening image in her mind of what nursing homes are like. Filthy hallways, horrid food, crazy people wandering about. Incompetent doctors and sadistic nurses. No privacy. No dignity. Left to die alone.

Chances are, your loved one has a similar image in his or her mind. Maybe you do, too. But this image is inaccurate. It's based on myth, misperception, and stereotype. And if you or your loved one make decisions about late life health care based on myth and misperception, you're liable to make very bad decisions.

Let's take a look at these myths, and see where they're wrong.

Myth #1: Dementia is an expectable part of aging— especially in our eighties and beyond

Fact: Almost everyone shows some decline in motor skill and cognitive function in their seventies and eighties, but a relatively small percentage of older adults develop Alzheimer's disease or some other form of dementia. Studies show that about 12 percent of eighty-four-year-olds show significant symptoms of dementia; by age eighty-nine, that number rises to about 25 percent. Put another way, 75 percent of eighty-nine-year-olds do not have dementia.

Myth #2: Medicare covers most of the cost for in-home care

Fact: Medicare covers part of the cost of in-home nursing or therapy services for a brief period following hospitalization or treatment in a skilled nursing facility. However, Medicare isn't designed to pay for the kinds of in-home help many people need, such as assistance with bathing, dressing, cooking, or cleaning. These services are sometimes covered by long-term-care insurance, but it depends on the policy.

Myth #3: Assisted living provides round-the-clock access to medical care

Fact: Most assisted living facilities have a registered nurse on the premises to respond to residents' everyday medical needs, but there is rarely a "doctor in the house." Even in skilled nursing facilities, physicians may be available during the day and on-call after hours, but they are rarely in the facility 24/7. Nursing staff act as the physicians' eyes and ears and make the day-to-day judgment calls (that's why they call them nursing homes).

Myth #4: All nursing home residents are senile or demented

Fact: Just over half of the people in nursing homes (about 53 percent overall) have some form of dementia (significant impairment in thinking and memory). The rest of the residents are usually alert and oriented. Many nursing home residents continue to manage their property and finances, participate in hobbies and religious activities, and have an active social life.

Myth #5: Nursing home residents have few legal rights

Fact: Nursing home residents have the same legal rights as any other U.S. citizen. Unless their medical condition dictates otherwise, a nursing home resident may vote, drive, interact with whomever he or she wishes, own property, and bear arms (although guns are rarely stored on nursing home grounds). Residents also have a number of rights specifically related to the nursing home and its staff. (We discuss these in detail in Chapter 8.)

Myth #6: Nursing homes offer only basic care—no frills required

Fact: Nursing homes are required by law to offer a safe, homelike environment and to address a vast spectrum of resident needs. The key word here is *homelike*. Nursing homes must provide entertainment, social interaction, exercise, access to religious services, transportation off-grounds, and privacy for personal matters (including an active sex life for residents who wish one).

Myth #7: Once you enter hospice, there's only one way out: feet first

Fact: To be eligible for hospice care, a patient must be declared terminally ill by a physician—that is, in the doctor's judgment, that patient has fewer than six months to live. But doctors don't have a crystal ball, and it's not unusual to go beyond the six months or even to get better and return home (or to assisted living or a nursing home). People do get discharged from hospice—sometimes more than once.

DID YOU KNOW...

- The typical caregiver is a married woman between the ages of forty and sixty. About 55 percent of caregivers work full- or part-time, but the average caregiver still spends eighteen hours each week in caregiving activities. About 15 percent of caregivers take at least one unpaid leave from work to devote more time to caregiving
- Caregivers in the United States spend more than $2 billion each month to cover out-of-pocket caregiving expenses—more than $30 billion each year.
- Nearly 60 percent of caregivers report significant symptoms of depression. About 20 percent report health problems related to caregiver stress, and caregivers with serious illnesses are more likely to succumb to them than are non-caregivers.
- At this moment, there are approximately 1.6 million people residing in nursing homes across America. More than 40 percent of today's seniors will use a nursing home at some point.
- The average yearly cost of nursing home care in 2007 was more than $70,000. In or near large cities, the average cost was more than $100,000. The most exclusive nursing homes averaged more than $120,000 a year.
- The U.S. General Accounting Office estimates that nursing home costs will *triple* in the next twenty years.

Sources: American Health Care Association, National Alliance for Caregiving, National Center for Healthcare Statistics, National Council on Aging, U.S. General Accounting Office.

A Framework for Caregiving

Knowing what assisted living facilities and nursing homes are really like will help you make better decisions about your loved one's care, but remember: Accurate information is just one part of effective caregiving. Effective caregiving also requires a long-term plan—a framework that guides your thinking and helps you apply the information you've acquired.

Our framework for caregiving is based on six principles:

GET FINANCIAL AND LEGAL
DOCUMENTS IN ORDER...NOW!

Early planning is important in many areas but particularly with respect to financial and legal matters. If your loved one's financial affairs need organizing, talk to an accountant and a Certified Financial Planner as soon as possible. If your loved one has not yet drafted some key legal documents (such as a will and a living will), speak with an attorney experienced in elder law. We provide suggestions for organizing finances and legal materials in Chapter 6. If work remains in either of these areas, you should take a few minutes to familiarize yourself with this material—the sooner the better.

- Plan ahead
- Get advice
- Get others involved
- Keep colleagues informed
- Take care of yourself
- Put things in perspective

Let's see how these principles come into play during the caregiving process.

Plan ahead

It's tempting to avoid difficult issues, especially those related to health care and long-term financial planning. Resist this temptation. If you take a proactive approach, addressing difficult issues early in the game, you can prevent them from escalating into emergencies. Ill-planned, last-minute solutions to complex health and financial problems rarely work out well.

Get advice

If you don't understand something, ask. People who have already been through this can be a great source of advice and comfort. So join a support group. Talk to doctors, nurses, and mental health professionals. When legal and financial concerns arise, speak with an attorney, accountant, or financial planner. Contact your local agency on aging or one of the organizations listed at the end of this book. No one can be an expert in everything, but the wise caregiver knows what she doesn't know and seeks advice from those who do.

IMPORTANT CONTACT INFORMATION FOR CAREGIVERS

Toward the end of this book, we provide contact information for agencies and associations related to aging and eldercare. Here are some key resources you'll need right away. Keep these phone numbers handy, and if you're a frequent Internet user, you might want to bookmark some homepages as well. These web sites not only provide a wealth of valuable information, but most also list e-mail addresses for different departments within the organization.

Organization	Telephone	Homepage
American Association of Retired Persons (AARP)	800-424-3410	www.aarp.org
Elderweb (Eldercare Resources)	309-451-3319	www.elderweb.com
Family Caregiver Alliance	415-434-3388	www.caregiver.org
Joint Commission on the Accreditation of Healthcare Organizations	630-792-5800	www.jointcommission.org
Medicare	800-633-4227	www.medicare.gov
National Association for Homecare and Hospice	202-547-7424	www.nahc.org
National Council on Aging	202-479-1200	www.ncoa.org
Social Security Administration	800-772-1213	www.ssa.gov

Get others involved

Caregiving works best when the burden is shared. Brothers, sisters, nieces, nephews, co-workers, neighbors, friends—everybody can pitch in and do something, large or small. And don't be afraid to ask for help from a family member whose schedule seems full. We're *all* busy. You are, too. Those who want to make time will. Those who don't won't. But you'll never know unless you ask. Research shows that those who reach out to others tend to be healthier and happier than those who insist on going it alone. (The same is true of the care receiver: The ability to ask for help and use it effectively is associated with healthier, happier aging.)

Keep colleagues informed

You might feel strange sharing private concerns with your boss or co-workers, but by doing so you'll help your colleagues understand your situation, turning misperception ("Why is she always late these days?") into empathy and support. Besides, it's likely that at least some of your co-workers are also coping with the challenges of caregiving; you can share your insights and experiences. Don't make a difficult problem worse by leaving others in the dark.

Take care of yourself

If you neglect your own needs, you'll become stressed. You won't think clearly, and you'll make bad decisions. One key to good caregiving is to take good care of yourself, both physically and emotionally. We discuss a variety of proven stress management techniques in Chapter 2.

Put things in perspective

In the midst of a pressing health problem, it's easy to think like Patricia, convincing yourself that things are "falling apart" and will never get better. This kind of short-term thinking is a trap, and it won't help you or your loved one. Put things in perspective by recognizing that change—even loss—can help a person grow. Remember, too, that some people have been through situations even worse than the one you are going through now. They survived, and so will you.

TAKING CHARGE: PROACTIVE STRATEGIES FOR MINIMIZING COGNITIVE DECLINE

One advantage of being an informed caregiver is that you can use this information to care for yourself as well. In recent years researchers have made great progress in developing strategies to minimize cognitive decline before it occurs, and reduce one's risk of developing dementia later in life. Here are a few:

- *Aerobic exercise.* In addition to being a great stress-reliever (as we discuss in Chapter 2), aerobic exercise enriches the brain's supply of oxygen, minimizing neuron loss and helping preserve cognitive function.
- *Mental stimulation.* The old adage is true: Use it or lose it. Any challenging mental activity can be helpful here: chess, bridge, crossword puzzles, Sudoku...even video games. Studies show that the more mental stimulation we receive, the lower our chances of developing dementia.
- *Antioxidants.* These are chemicals that can help preserve memory by deactivating highly reactive molecules that damage brain tissue. Antioxidants are found in many different foods, but especially good sources are blueberries, cranberries, kidney beans, pinto beans, plums, and red apples.

2

When Someone You Love Just Can't Make It Alone: Signs and Symptoms, Strategies and Solutions

Carolyn and her mother looked forward to their weekly lunches together. For Carolyn, these visits were a chance to hear about the goings-on in her mother's life; for Marguerite, they were an opportunity to impress her daughter and even show off a bit. Carolyn's visit was the highlight of her mother's week, and each Tuesday morning Marguerite tidied up the house, bought fresh flowers, and prepared one of Carolyn's favorite meals—beef stroganoff, perhaps, or her famous four-cheese lasagna.

Two Tuesdays ago, something seemed different. Carolyn didn't say anything at the time—she didn't want to upset her mother—but the apartment just didn't look right. Marguerite had always been a meticulous housekeeper, but two weeks ago...well, it was just plain weird. Right beside the coffee table was a pile of dirt and dust, and next to that the dustpan and a pair of rubber gloves. It was if her mother had almost finished sweeping the apartment, but somehow forgot to complete the job.

Then last week, another strange thing happened. There was an odd, putrid smell throughout the apartment—like food gone bad or spoiled milk. Carolyn sat and wondered as they chatted before lunch, but her mother seemed unaware that anything was wrong.

When the phone rang, Carolyn slipped into the kitchen. The

odor of rotting food was overwhelming. She opened one cabinet, then another. Finally, she located the source of the smell: a five-day-old package of hamburger meat sitting atop the dessert plates. Carolyn swallowed hard and fought back the urge to be sick. She gingerly picked up the spoiled meat and dropped it in the trash. She carried the trash down the hall while her mother was still on the phone and said nothing about what she'd found.

During yesterday's visit, things were even worse. The apartment was in shambles: wet towels strewn on the living room rug, orange peels scattered on the floor near the refrigerator. When Carolyn opened the trash can, she found a pile of letters, all unopened, along with three unpaid bills—one marked "Past Due," another stamped "Final Notice."

After lunch, Carolyn asked her mother about the bills. Marguerite denied throwing them away—claimed they must have fallen off the counter while she was cleaning. When Carolyn pressed on, an edge crept into her mother's voice. What did she expect, for goodness sake? How clean was *her* house, anyway? Perfect? Spotless?

Carolyn went to bed early that night but slept little. She tossed and turned, wondering what to do. Finally, she decided. She'd insist they go see the doctor, together, to tell him what had happened. Her mother would resist the idea—Carolyn knew that—but what choice did she have? She dreaded having to confront her mother. She dreaded the fight that she knew would ensue.

When older adults have difficulties making it on their own, the problem is usually caused by one of three things: *injury, illness,* or *cognitive decline.* Certain types of injury (for example, a broken hip) are so debilitating that caring for oneself is impossible during the early stages of the recovery process. Illnesses such as glaucoma or diabetes interfere with self-care as well, because they destroy eyesight (in the case of glaucoma) or bring about a host of health problems that are difficult to manage alone (in the case of diabetes). Cognitive decline resulting from Alzheimer's disease or some other form of dementia makes living alone impossible: The memory loss and confusion that result from these conditions invariably lead to dangerous situations (such as forgetting a pot on the stove).

Injuries and illnesses happen to everyone, but how can we know when a loved one is no longer able to make it on his or her own? The answer lies not in the illness itself, but in the degree to which the illness causes *functional decline*—impairment in the skills necessary for independent living. The first signs of functional decline can be subtle (like misplaced pills) or obvious (like rotting meat in the kitchen cupboard). As a caregiver, you need to recognize these telltale signs of a worsening situation, so you can act on them appropriately.

Common Signs of Functional Decline

Here are the most common signs of functional decline in ill or aging people. If your loved one shows one or two of these signs, you should be concerned, and monitor the situation closely. If more than one or two of these things occur, it's time to take action. Be on the lookout for:

- Spoiled or improperly stored food
- Evidence that food has not been properly prepared (burned or grossly undercooked meat, charred or blackened pots and pans)
- Tasks begun, but not completed (for example, clothes left to mold in the washing machine)
- Difficulty communicating (for example, rambling conversation, inability to find words to express a thought)
- Repetitive questioning (along with an inability to remember your frequently repeated answer)
- Significant decline in the overall cleanliness of the home
- Evidence that a pet has not been properly cared for (empty water dish, filthy cat litter)
- Unpaid bills and unopened correspondence
- Uncharacteristic change in spending patterns (making a large number of purchases or refusing to purchase anything at all)
- Significant decline in personal hygiene (such as dirty clothing, body odor, sloppy shaving, or bizarre makeup)

- Urine or feces stains on clothing, floor, or furniture (including "wet spots" on upholstery)
- Inappropriate clothing (for example, a heavy coat in hot weather or shorts in the middle of winter)
- Persistent confusion about day of week or time of day
- Forgetting how to use familiar implements (like a key) or perform simple tasks (like opening a bottle of pills)
- Reports from friends and neighbors of strange behavior
- Instances of the person getting lost, especially if she can't find her way home from a familiar place
- Misusing medication (either over- or underdosing) or deviating substantially from a medication schedule (for example, taking three pills at once rather than one pill three times per day)

What Factors Contribute to Functional Decline?

What causes a person to lose the ability to cook, communicate, or manage her money? Why would a person who has long been meticulous in her personal hygiene suddenly stop bathing or brushing her teeth? Studies show that functional decline in older adults can usually be traced to one or more of the following factors.

Physical changes

As we age, we lose physical strength, stamina, balance, and muscle control. These changes can make the tasks of daily living a challenge. Laundry baskets begin to feel like boulders—too much to handle, especially when clothes are wet. A trip to the bathroom takes longer than it used to—accidents may result. Balance problems make stairways hazardous. Slowed reflexes make driving a car or using power tools downright dangerous.

Certain diseases can produce similar problems, even in younger people. Arthritic joints, shortness of breath from lung or heart problems, pain that has not been diagnosed or treated properly—any of these conditions can make movement difficult and independent living unmanageable.

ACTIVITIES OF DAILY LIVING

Signs of functional decline may indicate that a person can no longer carry out his or her *activities of daily living*, or *ADLs*. Health care professionals divide ADLs into two categories: basic and complex.

Basic ADLs are skills so important that without them, we could never survive on our own. They include:
- the ability to feed oneself
- the ability to use the bathroom appropriately
- the ability to maintain acceptable personal hygiene
- the ability to dress properly for current weather conditions

To live independently, a person must not only master the basic ADLs, but also the *complex ADLs* that many of us take for granted. Complex ADLs include:
- shopping
- cooking
- communicating effectively with others
- following directions
- taking medication appropriately
- managing money

The first signs that a person needs extra help usually involve some slippage in complex ADLs. Loss of basic ADLs comes later and indicates a greater degree of functional decline (and greater need for care). Marguerite—whose difficulties we discussed at the start of this chapter—is an example of a person who has started to show slippage in her complex ADLs but not yet in her basic ADLs.

Perceptual changes

The perceptual changes that come with age can contribute to functional decline:
- *Vision deficits.* As we age, we become farsighted, losing the ability to focus on small details. It's difficult to shave or apply makeup if you can't see your face clearly. It's hard to write a check if you can't see the numbers.
- *Hearing loss.* Decreased hearing can make telephone conversa-

tion nearly impossible and cause a person to miss all sorts of buzzers and alarms—even those intended as warnings.

- *Changes in smell and taste sensitivity.* Losses in smell and taste can cause a person to overlook the fact that food has spoiled or that a pot has boiled over on the stove.
- *Decreased sensitivity to touch.* Poor circulation or other complications of illness decrease temperature sensitivity, leading to burns from scalding sink or shower water. When touch (or "tactile") sensitivity decreases, scrapes and cuts may go unnoticed and become infected.

Cognitive changes

For the most part, the way we process information doesn't change as we age, but two things do occur. First, the *speed* with which we process information declines, especially in situations where a rapid response is required. Second, we lose the ability to *divide our attention* and carry out two or more tasks simultaneously (like holding a conversation while driving).

As discussed in Chapter 1, some age-related decline in cognitive processes is normal, especially as we move into our seventies and eighties. However, when Alzheimer's disease or some other form of dementia affects memory, problem-solving, and language processing skills, our ability to perform the tasks of daily living can deteriorate quickly. Driving becomes risky—even downright dangerous. Banking or shopping during busy times leads to miscalculations and errors. Tasks that must be performed in a certain precise sequence—cooking, for example—become an insurmountable challenge.

Psychological changes

As we age, we continue to use coping strategies that worked in the past, even when these strategies are no longer effective. Lifelong personality traits become exaggerated through a process known as *disinhibition*. Thus, a person who has always relied on others for advice can become unbearably clingy, pestering friends and family members almost constantly. A once-effective "take charge attitude" can deteriorate into irritable cantankerousness or argumentativeness.

Some age-related exaggeration of long-standing personality traits happens in almost everyone, but especially in people who are frightened or unhappy. In fact, the more scared or upset a person is, the more strongly he or she clings to

JUST WHAT IS ALZHEIMER'S DISEASE, ANYWAY?

Alzheimer's disease has been in the media so often that most of us are familiar with the term. More than four million adults in the U.S. suffer from this dreaded illness—about 1 out of every 70 people—and that number is sure to increase as the population ages. Here's what we know:

What causes Alzheimer's disease?

The exact cause of Alzheimer's disease is unknown, but a person's genetic makeup almost certainly plays some role. The disease results in loss of brain cells, producing the *amyloid plaques* (hardened brain tissue) and *neurofibrillary tangles* (twisted protein filaments) that are telltale signs of the illness. Modern neuroimaging techniques reveal decreases in neural activity throughout the brains of Alzheimer's patients.

How does Alzheimer's disease affect behavior?

The key behavioral symptoms of Alzheimer's disease include:

- *Memory loss.* Alzheimer's disease always results in progressive, debilitating memory loss. In the earliest stages of the disease, memory loss may be subtle, but as the disease continues, it becomes more extensive and widespread. Toward the end, the person can no longer recognize familiar people, places, objects, and symbols (like words).
- *Language processing deficits.* Alzheimer's patients gradually lose the ability to process language (including the ability to read, write, speak, and understand the speech of others).
- *Loss of higher intellectual functions.* As the disease progresses, Alzheimer's patients lose the ability to organize thoughts or execute a planned sequence of actions. Once-simple tasks become impossible: the person can no longer use a key, write a check, or turn on the TV.
- *Mood and personality changes.* Most people with Alzheimer's disease show changes in mood and personality. Irritability, aggressiveness, and exaggeration of long-standing personality traits ("disinhibition") are common.

Is there a cure?

Presently, there is no cure for Alzheimer's disease, but the symptoms can be managed with drugs and behavioral interventions. The illness may progress for up to twenty years (though six to eight years is more typical), and often the individual's physical health remains quite good until late in the disease process. Most Alzheimer's patients live in nursing homes during the latter stages of the illness.

old, familiar ways. Depression and anxiety—both common in older adults—can interfere with functioning and contribute to functional decline.

Distinguishing Temporary Decline from Long-Term Deterioration

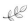

When is an accident merely an accident, and when is it a sign of a more serious problem? This can be hard to determine, because a single incident is usually not sufficient to confirm that functional decline is occurring. You have to look for a *pattern*—repeated incidents from the categories listed earlier. When problematic behaviors begin to repeat themselves or show up in a variety of areas, something is wrong. Do three things:

- Seek a diagnosis, and begin treatment
- Learn about the illness, and plan ahead
- Consider psychological factors

Seeking a diagnosis and beginning treatment

When a problem emerges, check first to see if an underlying illness is responsible (for example, glaucoma or diabetes). This requires a thorough assessment by a physician. If a medical problem is detected, the physician will recommend a course of treatment, and in many cases the problem behavior will disappear when the underlying cause is removed.

Learning about the illness and planning ahead

What if the problem is due to a medical condition for which there is no effective treatment? In such cases, the doctor may at least be able to predict the course of the illness, including a tentative time frame. Once you know what the problem is, you can gather information about it through textbooks, Internet sites, and national associations related to the illness (if they exist). Knowing what to expect helps you plan for the future.

Considering psychological factors

What if there's no medical basis for the problem behavior, or the behavior goes far beyond what usually results from the illness that's prompting it? Now you're looking at a problem behavior that is caused—at least in part—by psychological factors. In this situation, the problem should be addressed with psychotherapy, medication, and other behavioral interventions. The doctor should refer the patient to a psychologist or psychiatrist experienced in care of the elderly.

Getting Your Loved One to See the Doctor

Most people are willing to see their physician, as long as the two of them have a good relationship to begin with. However, if your loved one is the type that avoids doctors like the plague, you may have to do some persuading, coaxing, or cajoling. Several strategies are useful here:

- *Make the situation less frightening.* People born seventy or eighty years ago often learned to associate physicians with death, since people only saw the doctor when everything else had failed. Address this fear by reminding the person that medicine has advanced, and things have changed since they were young. Prepare them for what will happen in the office (who will be there, who does what, etc.); knowing what to expect can lessen anxiety. Finally, remind them of their rights as a consumer of health services, including their right to get clear explanations of all diagnoses and treatments, and to refuse treatment if they so choose.
- *Reframe the situation.* Many of us were raised to perceive doctors as infallible beings whose opinion is never questioned. Help your loved one view the doctor as a consultant or advisor, reminding him or her that all treatment decisions will be made in conjunction with the physician. Reframing the situation in this way will help the prospective patient feel more powerful and in control.
- *Enlist the help of others.* If your sister or your aunt or some other family member is a more effective nudge than you are, ask one of them to use their skills here. If Dad is more likely to do what his best friend or pastor suggests, ask one of them to speak with

SOME KEY INSURANCE TERMS

Insurance is an integral part of today's eldercare system. If your loved one hasn't reviewed her insurance situation recently, this might be a good time to speak with an insurance advisor experienced in working with older adults. We discuss insurance issues in detail in Chapter 5, but here are some terms you need to know right away:

- *Medicare.* Medicare is a federally funded program administered by the Department of Health and Human Services and available to all Americans over age sixty-five. Medicare has four major components, known as Parts A, B, C, and D. Here are the basics:
  - Medicare Part A (available to everyone) covers inpatient care and some aspects of in-home care.
  - Medicare Part B (which is optional and requires a monthly premium) covers many outpatient services.
  - Medicare Part C (also known as Medicare Advantage Plan) is available through Medicare-approved private insurance companies, and combines Medicare Parts A and B (it sometimes includes prescription drug coverage as well, depending upon the plan one chooses).
  - Medicare Part D (which includes a variety of plans and varying levels of coverage and co-payment) covers prescription drug costs.

  Both Part A and Part B include deductibles and co-payments, and exclude certain services. Part D also includes deductibles and co-payments, and may exclude or limit certain medications (depending upon the plan). People often purchase *Medigap* insurance to cover these additional costs.
- *Medicaid.* Medicaid benefits (also known as *Medical Assistance* benefits) are funded by federal, state, and local governments, and cover health care costs for low-income Americans. Medicaid will pay for some services rendered in hospitals or other certified health care institutions, but it rarely covers in-home care. To be eligible for Medicaid, you must meet stringent income and asset requirements.
- *Secondary insurance.* This is health care insurance, usually purchased privately, that is used to cover expenses not paid for by Medicare. Secondary insurance policies do not cover long-term health care costs, and rarely cover in-home care for an extended period.
- *Long-term-care insurance.* This form of insurance covers in-home and residential services (including nursing home services) over an extended period of time.

him about the importance of seeing the doctor. This may feel a bit sneaky, but sometimes it works.

As you can see, the idea here is to do whatever is necessary (within reason, of course) to get your loved one to the doctor's office. If possible, you should accompany him to his appointment so you can let the doctor know what you've observed. If you can't be there in person, communicate your concerns to the physician ahead of time. And if the doctor prefers to see the patient alone, don't argue. She might be able to get more information one-on-one than she could with you in the room.

Getting Your Loved One to See a Mental Health Professional

You thought getting Mom to see a doctor was tricky? Try getting her to see a psychologist. Many people are reluctant to see a mental health professional because of the stigma associated with mental illness, or, less often, because they are afraid of what the psychologist might find out about them. Older adults—who grew up in an era when few people spoke openly about mental health problems—can be particularly resistant to seeking help from a mental health professional.

If the physician recommends that a psychologist or psychiatrist be brought in, you'll need to confront this resistance head-on. The physician may be able to help, but in most cases the burden will fall on you to convince your loved one to follow through with the appointment. Here are the kinds of objections you're likely to hear, along with suggestions for countering these objections.

- *Shrinks are for crazy people.* Statistics might not help here (though more than 20 million Americans each year seek help from a mental health professional). Better to remind your loved one of people he respects who have sought treatment for mental health problems—a friend or relative, perhaps, or even a well-known media figure. Mike Wallace, Oprah Winfrey, Brooke Shields, Tipper Gore, Betty Ford, Patty Duke Astin, and many other celebrities have shared their treatment experiences, making it more acceptable for the rest of us to do the same.

- *I don't believe in that therapy mumbo-jumbo.* This objection can be countered by reminding your loved one that she is not in fact going for therapy. She's seeking an *evaluation*—an assessment of the situation by a qualified professional. This person might recommend treatment, but that's something the two of you can deal with down the line (and it's not a good idea to bring it up at this juncture unless your loved one raises the issue).

- *It's a waste of time.* That's an easy one: Let the person know he or she is worth the time, and that the two of you have nothing to lose by pursuing this option. You might get to the bottom of the problem, and if not, what have you lost? An afternoon, at most.

- *It's too expensive.* Another easy one: If the physician has deemed a psychological or psychiatric evaluation medically necessary, the services should be Medicare eligible. Coverage varies from state to state, but in most cases, Medicare will cover between 50 and 80 percent of the cost of an initial evaluation, as long as it is done by an approved provider. Much—or all—of the fee not covered by Medicare may be covered by the patient's secondary insurance.

- *They'll put me away.* This is a toughie, because the fact is, they might. If the problem is severe enough, the person might need inpatient psychiatric treatment or nursing home care. It's tempting to give false reassurance at this point, but don't. You'll lose your loved one's trust forever if she discovers you've misled her. Instead, emphasize that inpatient treatment is just that—treatment, not a prison sentence—and in most cases it's time-limited.

The Emotional Side of Caregiving: Changing Roles

One of the difficulties of caregiving is that it requires you and your loved one to find new roles within a long-standing relationship. After forty, fifty, or eighty

THE FAMILY AND MEDICAL LEAVE ACT

The 1993 Family and Medical Leave Act has been a blessing for working caregivers. The Act outlines a number of very specific caregiver rights and employer responsibilities. These include:

- A minimum of twelve weeks unpaid leave to care for an ill parent, spouse, or child (but not a grandparent or in-law).
- Flexibility in how the leave is structured: It can be taken all at once or a little at a time (though your employer can require that vacation and sick days be "spent" at the start of the leave).
- Continuation of employee health benefits during the leave (though you may have to reimburse your employer for this coverage if you do not return to work following the leave).
- Reinstatement in your old job, or one with equivalent pay, duties, and benefits (this right does not hold for employees who are among the 10 percent highest paid at the organization).

To fall under the protection of the Family and Medical Leave Act, you must be at an organization with fifty or more employees, and you must have worked for the company for at least one year (1,250 hours minimum). You should check with your company's personnel office as soon as possible if you're planning to request a leave. Different companies have different policies, and the Act requires that employees give thirty days advance notice of their intention to take a leave, if circumstances permit.

years together, this can be difficult. Let's look at these role changes from three different caregiver perspectives.

The adult child's perspective

In the majority of cases, the primary caregiver is an adult child of an aging parent. These are the most widely studied—and best understood—caregiver–care receiver relationships.

- *Parenting the parent.* After a lifetime of seeing your parent in a certain way, it can be difficult to accept that things have changed. The toughest of these changes involves a disturbing kind of role-reversal: Now, instead of being looked after by your parent, you're the decision-maker. Practice makes the task a bit easier, but many people never feel quite natural in their new role.

- *Emergence of mortality issues.* When your parents grow old or ill, their mortality becomes hard to ignore. And when your parents are gone, you're next in line. Frailty and illness in a parent is a very frightening thing. Not only are they mortal, but you are, too.

- *Old resentments re-emerge.* Parent-child relationships are extremely complex. Even the most loving relationships have bumps along the way: mistakes, misunderstandings, missed opportunities, and let-downs. If you've always harbored hidden resentment because Dad wouldn't let you apply to medical school, there's a good chance this resentment will re-emerge now that you're Dad's caregiver. You may find it useful to acknowledge these feelings during the caregiving process (though not everyone does or should). Whatever path you choose, be aware that old hurts still affect you. It's dishonest and unwise to pretend they don't.

The spouse's perspective

Oftentimes a spouse—usually the wife—is primary caregiver. When this is the case, a whole different set of challenges ensue.

- *A new kind of intimacy.* You've lived with someone for fifty years without ever having seen him in the shower. How would you feel about having to help him to the toilet every day and clean him up after accidents? It's often uncomfortable to perform caregiving tasks for a spouse, but it helps if you see it as an opportunity to create a new kind of intimacy that complements—but doesn't replace—the intimacy you've built up over the years. If you truly care about a person, you must get beyond the natural aversion most of us have to helping that person perform basic bodily functions.

CAREGIVER SUPPORT GROUPS

Support groups can be a very effective way of managing stress. They provide a source of information and comfort, an outlet for venting frustrations, and the reassurance of knowing that you're not in this alone. There are a variety of support groups out there, ranging from the specific (groups for caregivers of Alzheimer's or stroke patients), to the general (Children of Aging Parents). Some groups are led by a therapist or social worker; others are self-help ("leaderless") groups organized and run by the members themselves. You can obtain information regarding support groups in your area from local nursing homes and agencies on aging, or from any of the following associations.

Alliance for Children and Families
11700 West Lake Park Drive
Milwaukee, WI 53224
414-359-1040
www.alliance1.org

Family Caregiver Alliance
180 Montgomery Street, Suite 1100
San Francisco, CA 94104
800-445-8106, 415-434-3388
www.caregiver.org

National Alliance for Caregiving
4720 Montgomery Lane, 5th Floor
Bethesda, MD 20814
www.caregiving.org

- *Same old song.* If you're the jealous type, and your husband is now being cared for by half a dozen young nurses and aides, it's not going to sit well with you. If you've always seen your wife as a spendthrift, and she's now running up substantial medical bills, you're going to get upset. Old fears and worries won't go away during the caregiving process. They might even get worse, because they provide a "safe" way of expressing concerns about other scarier things like illness and death.
- *End of sexuality?* If you've remained sexually active throughout your marriage, but illness now prevents one or both of you from

being able to enjoy it, what do you do? Give it up? Find someone else? Should you continue to be intimate if your spouse no longer recognizes you? Age and illness bring up troubling questions with no easy, ready answers. It helps if the two of you discuss these issues openly and as early as possible during the caregiving process.

The sibling's perspective

Increasingly, the role of caregiver is assumed by a sibling. In other cases, two or more siblings share caregiving responsibilities for a parent. Both arrangements present certain challenges.

- *Now's your chance.* If you've always resented your brother's looks, his great job, and his lovely wife, congratulations: Finally, you've got the upper hand. If you've been waiting sixty years to get back at your sister for stealing your boyfriend in ninth grade, guess what? Now's your chance. Old hurts linger, and they can have an adverse impact on the caregiving process. If you suspect the decisions you're making about your sibling's care are being influenced by old, unresolved issues, talk to someone—anyone—about it. Talking about it will help put things in perspective.
- *Sibling rivalry resurfaces.* If you and your sister have spent your entire lives competing for Dad's approval, you can bet these old rivalries are going to resurface during caregiving. After all, he really needs you now, and it's your last chance to prove you really are the better kid.
- *Secret, shameful joy.* When we harbor unexpressed resentment toward a sibling who's now ill, we may find ourselves taking secret, shameful joy in his or her plight. Rest assured, this is normal. But you still have a responsibility to be a good caregiver, if that is the role you've accepted. Remember: Feelings are feelings, and they're neither good nor bad. Where caregiving is concerned, it's our actions that count—it's what we do, not how we feel while we're doing it.

Caregiver Stress and Its Effects

Health problems in someone you care about—especially serious health problems—affect you as well. They frazzle your nerves, muddle your thoughts, and wear you down, both physically and emotionally. Good caregiving involves coping effectively with caregiver stress. It means taking care of yourself so you can take better care of your loved one.

EMOTIONAL REACTIONS TO CAREGIVING: FOREWARNED IS FOREARMED....

No matter what your relationship to the care receiver might be—partner, sibling, daughter, son, or friend—some feelings are common to all caregivers. Expect to feel at least some of these things, and know that these feelings are a normal part of caregiving:

- *Anger.* Especially if the care receiver is a family member, it's easy to become angry, and wonder: Why us?
- *Guilt.* It's normal to think, Could I have done something to prevent this from happening? Let guilt come, then let it go. Dwelling on these questions won't do any good now. Your job is to focus on the task at hand: being the best caregiver you can be.
- *Sadness.* Serious health problems in someone close to us set in motion a kind of mourning process and nostalgia for past times when things were better.
- *Fear.* Caregiving is frightening—a leap into uncharted waters. Everyone feels overwhelmed and worries that they're not up to the challenge, especially early on in the process. (That's why you're reading this book: to help make an overwhelming task a bit less overwhelming.)

Physicians and psychologists divide the symptoms of caregiver stress into three categories. If you have six or more of these symptoms, including at least one symptom in each category, you are experiencing caregiver stress that might well interfere with your ability to function effectively:

Emotional signs

- Persistent feelings of sadness or depression

- Feelings of helplessness and hopelessness
- Frequent crying or tearfulness
- Anger, irritability, or decreased frustration tolerance
- Chronic anxiety
- Feelings of detachment—feeling cut off from others
- Feelings of unreality ("this isn't really happening")
- Loss of interest in pleasurable activities (including sex)
- Rapid shifts from one emotional state to another

Physical symptoms

- Decreased energy, easily fatigued
- Increased muscle tension
- Restlessness, jumpiness, difficulty sitting still
- Hyperarousal (startling easily)
- Shortness of breath or difficulty breathing deeply
- Rapid heartbeat ("palpitations")
- Heartburn and gastric distress (diarrhea or constipation)
- Difficulty becoming sexually aroused
- Headaches, tooth-grinding, muscle pain (such as a sore back or stiff neck)

Cognitive signs

- Difficulty concentrating, distractibility
- Difficulty organizing your thoughts
- Decreased attention span
- Memory problems (especially short-term memory)
- Preoccupation with real or imagined mistakes
- A newfound preference for sadistic or hurtful humor
- Obsessing and ruminating about negative things
- Diminished problem-solving ability
- Difficulty making decisions about simple matters

Coping with Stress Before It Overwhelms You

Caregiver stress is unavoidable, but it need not overwhelm you. Here are some things you can do to cope with stress before it gets out of hand:

SOCIAL SUPPORT, DISCLOSURE, AND HEALTH

How important is it to share your feelings with someone when you're going through difficult times? Consider:

- Illness and mortality rates are 30 percent lower in widows and widowers who share their grief with others than in those who try to "go it alone."
- Cancer patients who have high levels of social support live significantly longer than socially isolated patients, and they experience less pain and anxiety.
- Caregivers of Alzheimer's patients get sick less often when they talk to others about how they feel; those caregivers who share the most get sick the least (and they have the mildest bouts of illness).

The bottom line: Unburdening yourself is good for you, so talk about your feelings. You'll be healthier as a result—and a better caregiver as well.

- *Take time for yourself.* Caregiving is so demanding that caregivers often forget to take care of themselves. Remember to eat well, get enough sleep, and take time off to "recharge your batteries." Whether it's shopping, visiting with friends, walking your dog, or taking a bubble bath, set aside some time each day to do what you like. During this personal time, try not to think about caregiving responsibilities—no matter how pressing they may be. You might feel guilty indulging yourself when someone needs you, but do it anyway.
- *Look to others for support.* Caregiving is an enormous burden, and no matter how strong you are, you can't do it alone. Lean on others now and then, and let them offer support. Other people can listen, run errands, spend an afternoon with your kids, advise you, coach you, pat you on the back, or take you to dinner. Figure out what you need from those around you, and ask for it.
- *Unburden yourself.* Caregiving brings up a lot of feelings, many of them unpleasant. Studies show that sharing troubling feelings is one of the best ways of taming them. Find someone you trust, and tell that person how you feel. Unburden yourself. Whether

it's a friend, therapist, pastor, or Internet pal, let him know what you're going through. If you let it out, you'll feel better.

- *Simplify your life.* If there are other stressors in your life, consider putting them on hold or cutting them loose. Now is not the time to change jobs or go for that big promotion. New responsibilities may have to wait until this one is under control.
- *Exercise.* The findings are clear: Aerobic exercise (exercise that raises your heart and breathing rate) causes the brain to release stress-reducing, mood-enhancing chemicals. Find a way to build regular exercise into each week's schedule. Walk, play ball, do Pilates or t'ai chi—whatever pleases you. The important thing is to find something you enjoy and to do it regularly (but always check with your doctor before beginning a new exercise regimen).
- *Avoid alcohol and drugs.* Self-medication can be tempting, but it makes things worse in the long run. If you find yourself using alcohol or other drugs to "unwind" from the pressures of caregiving, you're at risk for developing a drug or alcohol dependence. If you really feel that you can't manage without a chemical boost, see your physician.
- *Hire a professional caregiver.* This might feel like "throwing in the towel," but sometimes a professional caregiver is just what's needed. It doesn't mean you're abrogating your responsibility; it means you're doing the best job you can to provide for your loved one. Finding a good caregiver is not a simple process, but it can be done. In Chapter 3, we'll show you how to find and fund good in-home care.

3

In-Home Care: Autonomy, Continuity, and a Bit of Extra Help

James breathed a sigh of relief when the phone call came. It had been a dogfight, but finally—*finally*—he had obtained funding for his wife to have in-home care three days each week. Since her stroke, Beatrice had been unable to look after herself, and while James did the best he could, he simply wasn't able to manage a full-time job along with caring for his wife.

When the home-care worker, Kathleen, arrived the first day, everything seemed fine. She showed up on time and seemed to know what she was doing. She'd worked with stroke patients before, she explained, and the worst thing the spouse could do was interfere. Let her do her job, she said, and after half an hour, she shooed James out the door. Not to worry, Kathleen assured him, Beatrice is in good hands.

After lunch that day, James called to see how things were going. There was no answer. He tried again, thinking he must have dialed the wrong number. Again, no answer. He waited and tried again ten minutes later. This time Kathleen picked up the phone. She'd been busy, she explained, helping Beatrice get dressed. But all was well, not to worry, Beatrice was fine.

Things went smoothly for the first couple of weeks. Sure, Beatrice complained about Kathleen—said she was snippy sometimes, and didn't always come when called. James became uncomfortable as he heard his wife's complaints. On the other hand, Beatrice could be demanding at the best of times, even when she was feeling good. And nowadays she complained about everyone and everything: doctors, nurses, noisy neighbors, garbage trucks, kids playing in the street. James figured Beatrice was just angry at being housebound and frustrated by the problems that resulted from her stroke.

Things got busy at work, and James was more grateful than ever for Kathleen's presence. Beatrice continued to complain, but for the most part, things seemed all right. James called on occasion, and usually someone answered. When they didn't, he called again, and eventually they picked up. If he could just get through the busy season, he'd have more time to spend with his wife. Just a few more weeks, and work would quiet down.

Ten days later the phone rang at work. James picked it up, and heard Kathleen's panicked voice. Beatrice had passed out. She fell in the bedroom and Kathleen couldn't lift her. The ambulance had just left and was on its way to the hospital.

When James arrived he got the news: Beatrice had suffered another stroke. It was much worse this time, and they didn't know if she'd pull through. James waited and worried. He felt terribly guilty that he hadn't been there. Maybe if he hadn't been so selfish, this wouldn't have happened.

In the end Beatrice did pull through, but the second stroke was a bad one, and Beatrice could no longer walk. She had trouble sitting upright now and couldn't chew or swallow. In-home care was no longer an option, and Beatrice was moved to a long-term care facility—a nursing home.

It took a lot of digging, but eventually James found out what happened. Kathleen, it turned out, had been watching TV, and she failed to hear Beatrice's cries through the closed bedroom door. Kathleen had forgotten to administer Beatrice's noon medication, and this time the consequences were disastrous: rising blood pressure, a burst artery, another stroke. Beatrice spent the rest of her life in the nursing home. She never came home again.

How could this have happened? Was James at fault? Is there anything he might have done differently that would have led to a more positive outcome?

Although James was well-intentioned, he made four mistakes that allowed a difficult situation to escalate into a crisis:

- He ignored key warning signs of a poor home-care worker.
- He didn't take his wife's complaints seriously enough.
- He didn't trust his instincts.
- He allowed work-related stress to cloud his thinking.

In this chapter, we explore the key elements of in-home care: finding and funding it, evaluating its quality, and dealing with problems that arise during the home care process.

Finding and Funding Good In-Home Care

There are many different types of home care services, and they vary according to the care-receiver's needs. The more complex the problem, the more highly trained the caregiver must be and the higher the cost. In 2007, the average cost per visit for a home care nurse was more than $120; the average cost per visit for a home health aide was more than $70.

To be covered by Medicare, a service must be ordered by the patient's physician, who declares the service *medically necessary*. A wide range of in-home services can fall into this category, including:

- Skilled nursing care
- Speech, physical, and occupational therapy
- Dietary and nutritional consultations
- Some educational services (for example, diabetes self-care)
- Rental or purchase of medical equipment (such as a wheelchair or blood-glucose monitor)

Keep two things in mind as you work out your plan for funding in-home care. First, in most cases Medicare will pay for in-home services only if the person has already been treated for the condition in a hospital or skilled nursing facility. Second, regardless of the severity of the problem, Medicare generally will not pay for *custodial care* (basic personal care such as bathing, feeding, toileting, and dressing).

How can you fund services not covered by Medicare? For many people, the best option may be a long-term-care insurance policy. Unlike Medicare, most long-term-care policies cover some custodial or nonskilled services (such as light housekeeping and transportation). Eligibility criteria (which often include waiting periods and dollar amount exclusions) differ from policy to policy; you should check with your insurer for details *before* you contract for services or file for benefits. (We discuss the basics of long-term care insurance in Chapter 5.)

Who May Provide In-Home Care?

In-home care is typically provided by certified home health care agencies and certified independent in-home caregivers, also known as *independent providers*.

WHO FUNDS IN-HOME CARE?

Costs for four-day-a-week in-home care averaged more than $20,000 per year in 2007, and a sizeable portion of these costs must be paid out of pocket. The good news is, if you hire a home care worker to care for an aging parent while you work, you may be able to obtain tax credits for up to 30 percent of the cost of the service. For up-to-date information on the latest regulations in this area, contact the Internal Revenue Service by phone at 800-829-1040 or online at www.irs.gov.

CHECKING UP ON AN AGENCY

Here are two good sources of information on a home health agency's accreditation status (including any past violations or pending investigations):

Joint Commission on Accreditation of Healthcare Organizations
One Renaissance Boulevard
Oakbrook Terrace, IL 60181
630-792-5000
www.jointcommission.org

National Association for Home Care and Hospice
228 7th Street SE
Washington, DC 20003
202-547-7424
www.nahc.org

Certified home health care agencies

A certified home health care agency is a corporation that provides a range of in-home health care services. To become certified, the agency must meet stringent federal and state standards in a variety of areas. The agency must also show that it adheres to all federal and state laws related to caregiving, patients' rights, storage and handling of medical information, and use of public and private funds.

Certified agencies must make their customer satisfaction data (ratings by past care recipients and their families) available to anyone who requests it. Don't be shy about asking for this information: Reputable agencies are usually happy to share it with you. In fact, if you ever encounter resistance when you request information in this area, consider it a warning sign. The agency may well be hiding something and should probably be avoided.

Certified home health care agencies can be found through many sources. These include:

• The patient's physician (who is probably familiar with most of the local options)

- The local Medicare office (which can tell you if an agency is eligible to provide a covered service)
- The office of the patient's private insurer
- The local chapter of the Visiting Nurses Association of America (its nationwide office number is 800-426-2547)
- Area hospitals, nursing centers, and social service agencies
- The National Association for Home Care (202-547-7424 or www.nahc.org)

Be forewarned: A certified home health care agency can be a rather formal operation, with a fair amount of red tape. Forms must be filled out, documentation provided, and so forth. These things may seem like hurdles, but they are really intended as safeguards. For example, when you provide an agency with your loved one's secondary insurance numbers, the agency can determine exactly what services she's entitled to receive. Oftentimes, the agency's

---

SHOULD YOU EVER USE AN AGENCY THAT IS NOT CERTIFIED?

Because the process is lengthy and expensive, not all agencies are certified. A fledgling home care agency might not yet have the equipment needed to meet federal and state guidelines, but in some cases they can still offer reliable, professional service. Agencies that are not certified usually offer their services at lower cost, since they don't have to pay the more highly-trained staff required by certification guidelines.

If all your loved one needs is a dependable, pleasant companion to provide supervision and some light housekeeping, an uncertified home care agency might be an appropriate option. However, remember that an uncertified agency isn't operating under the watchful eye of federal and state reviewers, and they need not screen or monitor staff as carefully as a certified agency does. If you use an uncertified home care agency, be especially vigilant for signs of poor care.

groundwork will enable the patient to get access to benefits you didn't know existed—and better care as a result.

Another advantage of working with an agency is that in the long run, the agency can reduce your paperwork burden considerably. They do the billing and recordkeeping for you, and since they deal with these matters every day, they get pretty good at fighting through insurance and government roadblocks that would leave most of us tearing our hair out.

Independent providers

Not all good caregivers choose to work for agencies. Many prefer to offer their services privately, deciding for whom they will work on a case-by-case basis. Independent providers of home health care can usually be located through Medicare, other third party payors (insurance companies), or the Yellow Pages. (Look under "Home Health Services" and "Nurses.")

Like home health care agencies, independent providers are required to meet certain criteria in order to be licensed. They must have adequate training and appropriate experience. They must also have malpractice insurance, adhere to the ethical standards of their profession, and fulfill continuing education requirements to stay up-to-date on the latest findings and treatments.

FAMILY MEMBER AS CAREGIVER (AND PAID FOR IT!)

There's an interesting "loophole" in many long-term care insurance policies: Although most policies require that custodial and nonskilled care be provided by persons who have completed formal training, some policies will actually pay for family members to get this training, and then reimburse them for the services they render. In other words, it may be possible for you to get paid for providing care to a family member, as long as your policy covers this and you meet the policy's eligibility criteria. The advantage for the insurance company is that they save money (since you'll be reimbursed at a lower rate than a more highly trained provider). The advantage for you is that you'll know your loved one is getting top-notch care (since you'll be the one providing it).

The independent provider is required to do all these things, but do they? Usually, but not always. If you use an independent provider, be prepared to investigate their background and credentials thoroughly. Most independent providers are legitimate, but as in every profession, there are some charlatans out there. Be wary, and investigate a potential home care provider thoroughly *before* you contract for services.

Remember, too, that no matter how skilled or devoted an independent provider may be, he or she is still only one person. You can expect that at some point your independent provider will call in sick or need a personal day to take care of a family emergency. Needless to say, if Mom needs help getting to the bathroom, she won't be able to put her needs on hold until the caregiver returns on Thursday.

The bottom line: If you use an independent provider, you'll eventually need to arrange backup coverage. Many independent providers make their own backup arrangements, but don't assume this without asking. Raise the issue ahead of time, and make arrangements in advance.

How to Evaluate an Agency or Provider

Once you find an agency or independent provider, how do you assess the quality of their services? First, *meet with them personally*. There's nothing like a face-to-face interaction to help you judge a potential caregiver. Second, *review their references and credentials*. Everything should be in order here—no exceptions, no excuses. Third, *ask others about the provider's performance*. Past clients are a great source of input. Finally, *trust your instincts*. If something feels wrong, it probably is.

On page 235, we've provided a Home Health Care Comparison Checklist you can take with you when you begin the evaluation process. This checklist will ensure that you cover all the important issues. And don't be afraid of offending potential providers by asking questions or even showing them the checklist. Any good caregiver will welcome a thorough evaluation of his services. He'll be impressed that you did your homework and know you mean business.

Here's a quick summary of the topics you should cover in your evaluation:

Questions to ask the agency

- How long have you been in the area?
- Which doctors and hospitals do you work with most closely?
- Have you ever received service awards from federal and state overview boards?
- Have you ever been censured by a federal or state board?
- What are your customer satisfaction ratings?
- How do you recruit and reward good staff?
- Can you guarantee full staff coverage? How?
- What are your procedures for addressing complaints or problems?

Questions to ask the independent provider

- Were you trained at accredited institutions?
- Are you certified and/or licensed in your profession?
- To what professional groups or organizations do you belong?
- How long have you been doing this kind of work?
- Have you ever been accused or convicted of malpractice?
- Have you ever been censured?
- Have you received any awards or commendations for your work?
- Do you have experts to whom you can turn on short notice, should an emergency arise?

Questions to ask former clients and their families

- How reliable was the provider?
- How well did the provider communicate with you and the patient?
- Did you have any problems with the provider? What were they?
- Would you use this provider's services again?
- How well did the provider perform in an emergency?

Caregiver qualities you'll have to assess yourself

Questions are important, but not all information can be obtained just by asking. To evaluate a potential caregiver, you'll need to judge a few things for yourself. Any good caregiver—whether she is an independent provider or employed by an agency—should have six qualities:

- *A professional appearance.* Appearance provides clues about a person's attitude and commitment. Although most caregivers don't look like television nurses, a sloppy or unkempt appearance simply isn't acceptable. A professional caregiver should be clean and well-groomed, and dressed appropriately for the job. Try to not be put off by generational norms (blue hair or a pierced nose don't mean a person is a bad caregiver). And don't be fooled by size: Some overweight people move quickly and smoothly, and some smaller people are surprisingly strong, especially if they're well-trained and use the proper equipment.

- *Good observational skills.* Good caregivers are observant. They must be sensitive to changes in the patient's condition—especially those the patient can't describe directly. Observational skills are hard to evaluate in a brief interview, but having the caregiver interact with the care receiver can be helpful in this regard. Together, you and your loved one can judge whether the caregiver seems to have a "feel" for the situation and the skills needed to identify changes in the patient's physical and emotional states.

- *Good communication skills.* A caregiver must be able to communicate clearly with folks who have perceptual problems. Ironically, good communication skills can sometimes make a caregiver seem a bit odd on first meeting. After all, caregivers are accustomed to working with those who are hard of hearing, so they may speak slowly, loudly, and very directly. In normal conversation, we generally don't ask people if they need to use the bathroom, but for a caregiver, this is a pretty standard question, and one much appreciated by someone who can't verbalize their needs.

- *Quiet self-confidence.* Arrogance isn't helpful, but quiet self-confidence is essential in a caregiver. After all, part of the caregiver's job is to provide reassurance to you and your loved one. A good caregiver helps both patient and family member feel that everything is in good hands.

- *An open mind.* Caregivers and care receivers are often quite different—in age, gender, and perhaps religious or ethnic background as well. A good caregiver must be open-minded and tolerant of ideas and beliefs that might not be the same as hers. Care receivers often vent their frustration on those around them, blurting out insults (including racial epithets) when depressed or upset. An experienced caregiver expects this and won't take it personally.
- *A sense of humor.* Professional caregivers know to expect the unexpected. Their clients are often stressed and cranky. Food gets spilled. Bedclothes get soiled. An even temperament and a dose of good humor are essential in a caregiver whose work is sometimes unpleasant.

The Trial Period

Once you've judged a caregiver to be acceptable, it's a good idea to begin with a one- or two-week trial period. Partway through the trial period, ask the care receiver how she feels about the caregiver. Ask her to evaluate the caregiver in specific, concrete areas—quickness of response, patience, gentleness, professional manner, and so forth. It's important that the care receiver feel comfortable with the caregiver, but *competence* is the essential ingredient here. A pleasant but incompetent caregiver can do more harm than good.

Agencies usually offer more flexibility than individual caregivers when it comes to caregiver-patient fit. Good agencies know that not everyone can work well together and that the first match-up might not be the one that sticks. Most agencies will allow the patient to work with several different caregivers in trial runs, if need be. Working with an agency doesn't ensure that you'll get your first choice of caregiver, but you should be able to specify your preferences, and the agency should make a reasonable effort to match you with someone you like.

Here we see another advantage of an agency over an independent provider. If you reject an agency caregiver, she'll probably get another posting right away—no hard feelings. On the other hand, if you reject an independent

THE GERIATRIC CARE MANAGER

In recent years, a new eldercare specialist has arrived on the scene—the *Geriatric Care Manager* (sometimes called a *Case Manager*). Geriatric Care Managers are usually nurses or social workers with training and experience in eldercare. They can help arrange home health care, nursing home placement, and a variety of other services. Geriatric Care Managers also coordinate different aspects of care, monitor progress, and oversee transfers among different care settings. Because they are usually well-connected within the area, Geriatric Care Managers can cut through a lot of red tape in a relatively short time. For the long-distance caregiver with a faraway loved one, the Geriatric Care Manager is especially helpful.

Geriatric Care Managers usually charge a flat fee of about $200 for the initial assessment, and an average hourly fee of about $75 for additional work. These fees are rarely covered by Medicare or private insurance, and it's a good idea to put fee arrangements in writing before you begin. Sometimes a local senior center will offer free or subsidized access to a Geriatric Care Manager on a short-term, time-limited basis.

You can locate Geriatric Care Managers through local senior centers and nursing homes. The National Association of Professional Geriatric Care Managers and the National Association of Social Workers also offer referrals and recommendations. They can be contacted as follows:

The National Association of Professional Geriatric Care Managers
1604 North Country Club Road
Tucson, AZ 85716
520-881-8008
www.caremanager.org

The National Academy of Social Workers
750 First Street NE, Suite 700
Washington, DC 20002
202-408-8600
www.naswdc.org

provider who happens to worship where you worship, or shop where you shop, you might have to deal with a rather awkward situation for a while.

When More Than One Person Needs Care

Many people caring for an ill or frail parent are surprised to discover that their healthier parent requires as much help and support as the identified patient—sometimes more. This is especially true if over the years the identified patient was primary manager of the household. After all, if one partner did all the cooking and cleaning during a fifty-year marriage, the other partner may not be able (or willing) to learn these skills now, especially with all the other changes taking place in their lives. These situations provide some real challenges for home care workers, who are rarely willing to provide "twofer" coverage when being paid to care for only one person. Hiring separate caregivers for Mom and Dad might seem like the ideal solution, but the presence of multiple caregivers in the home at the same time can lead to considerable chaos and conflict.

The bottom line: It's important to realize that the needs of the identified patient do not exist in a vacuum. In planning for in-home care, try to determine the needs of *all* members of the household when estimating how much coverage will be required. Most people underestimate how much help is needed, so err in the other direction. It's better to have too much help than too little, especially early on.

When Problems Arise During In-Home Care

The majority of caregivers are good and compassionate people, devoted to their patients' well-being. Some, however, are not.

Important warning signs of a poor home-care worker

At the start of this chapter, we described the problems experienced by James and his wife Beatrice as a result of a poor home-care worker. No matter how carefully you evaluate things ahead of time, it is impossible to predict with

RESPITE CARE

Hiring an in-home caregiver is not your only option. If your loved one does not need skilled nursing care, but you're still having trouble coping on your own, consider *respite care*, which can take several forms:

- *Informal caregiving arrangements.* If all that's needed is a pleasant companion who can do some light housekeeping, an informal caregiving arrangement with a trusted friend or neighbor may be appropriate. If you choose this option, take some precautions up front. Be sure both parties are clear on the caregiving expectations and financial arrangements. Put everything in writing. Leave a clear list of instructions (including medication and emergency contact information). And be prepared to terminate the arrangement if things don't work out (an awkward situation, but necessary if you're not satisfied with the service).

- *Temporary in-home care.* Home health care agencies and independent providers are often willing to provide in-home care on a time-limited, "as needed" basis. You can arrange for someone to provide care for a few hours, a day or two—whatever you need. This type of service is not covered by Medicare or most private insurance policies, but sometimes volunteers from local agencies and support groups will provide free short-term respite care. Contact your local Agency on Aging for a list of volunteer providers.

- *Overnighter options.* Many nursing homes, hospitals, and mental health centers offer overnight or weekend "getaway" programs for seniors in need of limited nursing care. Once the patient is deemed eligible by a physician, he or she can schedule a night or weekend "sleepover." Sleepovers enable caregivers to attend after-hours work-related events and can be used to provide the caregiver with some "time off" from caregiving. Limited emergency coverage is available in most overnighter programs.

100 percent accuracy how someone will perform in the future. Here are some important warning signs of a poor home-care worker:

- Unanswered phone calls or a constant busy signal
- Television or radio remaining on throughout the day
- Late arrivals, early departures, last-minute cancellations
- Health care equipment (needles, swabs, etc.) in the trash, instead of properly disposed
- Significant decline in the cleanliness of the home
- Evidence of illegal drugs in the home (for example, lingering odor of marijuana)
- Signs that the caregiver has been drinking alcohol while on the job or before arriving for work (for example, alcohol on the caregiver's breath)
- Presence of other people in the home (for example, unexplained visitors, the home-care worker's children)
- Frequent complaints on the part of the care receiver
- A troubling change in the care receiver's behavior (for example, increased depression, agitation, or confusion)
- Reports from neighbors that something is awry
- *Any* sign—no matter how "minor"—that abuse, neglect, or exploitation has taken place (these signs are described in detail below)

Confronting a poor caregiver

It is important that you confront a caregiver when you suspect something's wrong, but the *way* you confront the caregiver is critical. Be tactful but firm. Try not to sound accusatory or blaming, but express your concerns clearly and directly. Ask specific questions about the care receiver's concerns, as well as your own. Don't mince words. Ask questions until you're completely satisfied with the answers. If something needs to be changed, continue the discussion until you've developed a mutually agreed-upon plan of action. Set a follow-up meeting to assess how well the changes are working. And if, after you've pressed the issue, you conclude that something *is* wrong and it can't be fixed, do three things:

- Document the problem—take detailed notes describing the problem, photographs if necessary.
- Terminate the service, and begin the process of obtaining replacement service.
- Report your suspicions to the home health care agency if the caregiver is an agency employee, or the appropriate state licensure/certification board if the caregiver is an independent provider.

Signs of Abuse, Neglect, or Exploitation

Poor caregiving is bad enough, but the following signs and symptoms may indicate that abuse, neglect, or exploitation of the care receiver has taken place—a very serious situation. These signs must *always* be taken seriously. Never, *ever* ignore:

Physical symptoms

- Bruises, fractures, burns, or "impossible" injuries (for example, a dislocated elbow in a bedfast patient)
- Evidence of dehydration or malnutrition
- Exposure injuries (for example, hypothermia)
- Signs of improper medication

Psychological symptoms

- Hypervigilance ("hyper-alertness") on the part of the care receiver
- Undue concern with "what [the caregiver] wants"
- Development of new phobias and fears
- Persistent signs of upset prior to caregiver arrival (for example, pleading with you not to leave)

Financial signs

- Unexplained withdrawals from checking or savings accounts
- Appearance or disappearance of valuable items

WHEN THE ABUSER IS A FAMILY MEMBER

Sadly, most instances of physical, emotional, and sexual abuse are not perpetrated by strangers, but by family members. Abuse cuts across all financial, religious, and ethnic boundaries—don't assume your family is immune. Some people are deliberately hurtful, of course, and there are more than a few con artists out there just itching to take a trusting person's money. But most of the time, abusers are simply well-intentioned caregivers—people just like us—who were stressed beyond their limits and momentarily lost control.

If, in the course of caregiving, you find yourself yelling, threatening, handling your loved one roughly, or deliberately ignoring requests for assistance, *get help immediately*. Call a crisis intervention hotline, or contact a caregiver support group. It will be hard to admit what happened, but there's no shame in succumbing to stress. The shame is in not facing up to the problem and not doing something about it.

If you suspect that a friend or family member is abusing someone in their care, confront them calmly but directly, and insist they get help. Do not permit them to provide care until the problem has been addressed. Remember: *If you don't act to stop abuse, you are a party to the abuse—as guilty as the person doing it.* Failing to report abuse may even make you legally liable for future incidents, just as if you had committed them yourself.

- Evidence that unnecessary services have been ordered
- Changes in the care receiver's legal or financial status
- Unusual contributions to charities

Reporting Abuse, Neglect, or Exploitation

You have a moral obligation to report abuse, neglect, or exploitation if you observe it in a caregiver. Not only will you be protecting your loved one, but you'll be protecting other, future care receivers who might otherwise be harmed.

If you detect any of the signs listed earlier, don't delay. Take the three steps outlined in the previous section (*document the problem, terminate the service,* and *report your suspicions to the appropriate authority*). In addition, add a fourth step: Report your concerns to the local Elder Abuse program. Their telephone number should be listed in the "Human Services" section of the phone book, usually near the child and spouse abuse hotlines. You can find the telephone number of your state's Elder Abuse program through the Elderweb's Online Eldercare Sourcebook (www.elderweb.com). If you don't have Internet access, you can obtain contact information for reporting suspected abuse by calling 800-677-1116.

4

When In-Home Care Becomes Impossible: Screaming, Crying, Fighting...and Moving On

The three women chatted amiably, but Lucy could feel the tension in the air. Mom was nervous, defensive. She knew why they were there, and she kept up a steady stream of chatter that prevented her daughters from changing the subject. When the waiter arrived with the main course, the conversation slowed. Lucy saw her opening. It was time to begin.

"Mom," said Lucy gently, "we really need to talk."

Her mother's expression slowly changed. Her smile faded, and her shoulders sagged a bit. She gazed down at her plate.

"I...we...Irene and me, we think it might be time for you to move somewhere safer." Lucy looked at her mother, but there was no response. "Safer," she repeated, "and more comfortable."

After a brief pause, Lucy's mother spoke, so softly it was barely a whisper.

"You're putting me away?"

"Not putting you away, Mom. Arranging for you to be somewhere safe, where you can get the care you need."

"Just like that, you're putting me away?"

Irene spoke up. "Mom, it's not like that."

"What about the house? What about my cats?"

"We'll take care of everything, Mom. I promise."

"But I'm fine at home. It's all right. I'm OK."

"Mom, please. It's not all right. You know what's been happening. I mean, just last week…"

"You're going to tell me it's for my own good, right? Don't bother. I know why you're doing this. I've become too much trouble. Too big a burden."

Irene spoke up again. "Mom…"

"Enough!" Irene and Lucy flinched at the sound of their mother's angry voice. "Enough! I won't hear any more of this!"

There was silence for a moment—just the sound of other diners talking quietly in the background. Then a harsh command: "Irene, take me home."

Irene stood up, not knowing what to do or say. Lucy watched helplessly as her mother moved away from the table in tiny, shuffling steps. Irene hesitated, then followed. Suddenly, Mom turned to face them. Her eyes were full of fury, her body rigid with anger.

"You'll never get away with this. Mark my words. Never!" And with that, she moved through the doorway, and out of the restaurant. Then Irene was gone too, and Lucy was alone.

Lucy was afraid to look up, but she didn't really have to. She could feel the eyes of the other patrons staring at her in shock and disbelief. She knew what they were thinking—how could a daughter do this to her mother! Lucy sat quietly, thinking the very same thing.

Here's what we wish for when we meet with a loved one to discuss nursing home placement: heartfelt expressions of gratitude, and thanks for our hard work and thoughtfulness. In most cases, here's what we get: anger, tears, pleading, threats, insults, and slamming doors.

There's no easy way to raise the issue of nursing home placement with someone you love. In many ways it's the most difficult part of the entire nursing home process. In this chapter, we discuss strategies for tackling this challenge: talking about options with family members, raising the issue with the care receiver, and ensuring that your loved one gets adequate care even if she refuses all offers of help.

Talking About Options with Other Family Members

The first step in nursing home placement involves discussing the situation with those closest to the care receiver. These talks not only provide input from those who care most, but they also help build a consensus among people the care receiver loves and trusts. Since most care receivers are initially resistant to the idea of nursing home placement, a "united front" of family members is key to selling the idea.

Family discussions work best if you have a plan. Your plan should involve four steps: *beginning the discussion, exploring possibilities, building consensus*, and *turning thoughts into actions*.

Beginning the discussion

Before you meet as a group, talk with each person individually and find out how they view the situation. If your family is like most, you'll probably get a range of opinions—perhaps some wildly divergent views. By knowing how people feel ahead of time, you can anticipate the issues that will be raised and the kinds of conflicts that will arise during the discussion.

Keep the first meeting small, so it doesn't become chaotic. You can bring in others later, as needed. Immediate family—children, spouse, and siblings—should be involved in the initial discussion, but only include other family members if they have a unique relationship with the care receiver (for example, a cousin or niece who's especially close).

If not everyone can attend your first discussion, meet anyway. Time is of the essence where nursing home placement is concerned. If a face-to-face meeting is impossible, consider a conference call or an Internet chat meeting. Or gather as many key players as you can, and bring in the rest over a speakerphone.

Exploring possibilities

Open the meeting by reviewing the history of the situation—changes in your loved one's health or behavior, his present level of functioning, the likely progression of the illness during the next weeks or months. As you do this, focus on the person's present and future needs: What, exactly, does he need right now? What will he need six months from now? What can he do on his own today? Will that still be true in six months or a year?

WHEN YOU CAN'T CHOOSE THE TIME OR PLACE

All too often, discussions of important care decisions take place at midnight, with tired, stressed family members huddling in hospital corridors. Needless to say, this isn't an ideal setting for such an important decision. If a crisis situation dictates that you must hold a spur-of-the-moment "emergency meeting," try to find a more congenial setting. Ask staff if you can use an empty conference room, chapel, or lounge. If you're too tired to think straight, go get some coffee. If you need spiritual guidance, ask that the on-call pastor be paged. If you have questions for the doctor, ask to speak with her—and don't commit to anything until you've gotten the information you need.

Next, generate a list of possible solutions for the needs you've identified. Write them all down. It's OK to be a bit vague at this point—don't worry about the details just yet. Include in your list some ideas that might seem far-fetched or unrealistic. Inspiration often comes from unexpected places, and you're not committing yourself to anything right now.

When you're done brainstorming, take a short break. Give people a chance to catch their breath. Then reconvene, review your list, and rank the options from best to worst. Throw out the worst ideas, and focus on the two or three best options. Write each option on a separate index card, and generate a list of questions you'll need answered to make your decision about that option.

Now go out and get the information you need to answer those questions. Use the Internet and telephone contact information in the back of this book, or get in touch with local nursing homes and agencies on aging. And by all means, divide up the tasks so the entire burden doesn't fall on one person. Everyone should contribute to this initial information-gathering effort.

Building consensus

When you have the information you need to choose among your options, have a second meeting to make a final decision. Don't let too much time pass between these meetings; a day or two would be ideal—a week at the very most. You don't want to lose the momentum you gathered during your first meeting, and too long a delay will encourage people to procrastinate instead of gathering material right away.

Begin the second meeting by having each person summarize the information he or she obtained, then weigh different options. Summarize points of agreement out loud, then write them down. Try to be objective, and reflect the group's opinion, even if it conflicts with yours.

You might arrive at a unanimous decision right away. More likely, there will be one or two dissenters from the majority. Explore the dissenters' objections, and see if they can be convinced to go along with the group. Emotions may run high at this point, so be prepared to call "time out" if tempers flare. Let the discussion run its course, but don't end the meeting until a consensus has been reached that is acceptable to all the key players. Some compromise on everyone's part might be necessary to get to that point.

Turning thoughts into actions

Four steps are needed to accomplish this:

- *Speak with the care receiver's physician.* This is important, because the physician may be the only person familiar with the three key elements of the situation: the patient, the illness, and the local facilities. The physician is also responsible for determining when the patient meets the criteria for ADL deterioration that trigger the onset of insurance benefits (see page 14 for more information about ADLs). Ask the physician where your loved one stands with respect to his or her ADLs.

- *Consult with an attorney experienced in elder law.* This person can help you craft some crucial legal documents (for example, a health care proxy), that many nursing homes ask for at the time of admission. An attorney experienced in elder law can also advise you on state and federal laws regarding wills and estates, and on strategies for asset management. At this point, you might also want to speak with a financial consultant to get additional advice on how to safeguard your loved one's assets.

- *Set up appointments to visit local nursing homes.* Most nursing homes are glad to provide tours, meetings with staff, and written materials describing their services. Given some basic information about your loved one's insurance situation, nursing homes can sometimes estimate monthly out-of-pocket costs and advise you about funding options. Be sure to ask each nursing home whether they have a waiting list, and if so, how long it is: The best facilities can be harder to get into than Ivy League schools. Don't be put off by a nursing home with a long waiting list, but be advised that months—sometimes years—may pass before an opening arises. (There's no law that says a person can't start out in one nursing home and move to a more desirable one when a spot opens up.)

- *Speak with the care receiver's insurance company.* Medicare, Medicaid, and private insurers usually have regional offices staffed with people well-versed in coverage guidelines. You might feel as though you need a translator to understand what insurance officials are saying, but try not to be intimidated by unfamiliar terms. Persist, and ask questions until you're satisfied. You won't always be happy with what you hear, but don't blame the messenger. Insurers can be valuable allies if you take care not to alienate them.

Raising the Issue with the Care Receiver

Raising the prospect of nursing home placement with the care receiver is never easy or pleasant, and there's nothing we can do to change that. But by following a few guidelines, you can make the discussion go as smoothly as possible.

Who should participate?

To answer this question, you need to think about how the care receiver reacts in family situations. If you know from experience that this person is likely to be persuaded by a united front of family members, then raise the issue as a group. If you think the care receiver would be most receptive to one or two people, then those people should meet with the person privately.

Where should you meet?

Choose a meeting place where you'll have privacy and no interruptions. It should be a place where the care receiver feels safe and comfortable, such as her home or yours. Avoid intimidating settings like a doctor's office, and do not raise the issue in a public place like a restaurant. As Irene and Lucy found out the hard way, that's just asking for trouble.

When should you do it?

You might not have a lot of leeway here, particularly if the problems are pressing. If a group meeting is needed, it's likely that no time will be convenient for everyone; just do the best you can, and fill in the no-shows later. Whatever time you choose, make sure everyone clears his or her schedule. This is not an appropriate setting for people to take phone calls, check in with the kids, and so forth.

As you plan this meeting, remember that the care receiver has a schedule as well. Don't set a time that conflicts with her activities (for example, a favorite television program); if you do, she's likely to be late or miss the meeting entirely. And be prepared to meet more than once. You might get everything resolved in a single session, but sometimes it takes several tries to bring the care receiver on board.

THE BEST-LAID PLANS...AND SOME COMMON FAMILY ROADBLOCKS

Your family met, came up with a plan, and got Mom's tentative agreement. Then, just as you start to finalize the arrangements, things start to slip. Brother decides he can't contribute as much time as he'd promised. Sister can't cope with the house being sold. Your rarely-seen cousin surfaces and offers to move into Mom's place and care for her—as long as her three kids and two dogs can come along.

Suddenly, everyone has their own agenda. What's going on here? You did everything right, so why isn't your plan working?

It *is* working. These are normal responses as people come to grips with the full implications of their decisions. Don't get frustrated by your family members' inconsistency. Instead, understand the issues that are getting in the way:

- *Financial concerns.* Let's be honest: Some people perceive money spent on nursing home care as inheritance squandered. Sometimes this stems from genuine financial need, but at other times, people are struggling with fear of independence. Deep down they believe they can't make it on their own, and the fragility of a family member is bringing this to the surface, in the guise of a financial worry.

- *Overidentification.* Empathy is a fine thing: It helps us see the world as others see it and be sensitive to others' feelings. But sometimes empathy can turn into *projection*—a psychological process wherein we unconsciously "project" our own concerns into other peoples' heads. Statements like, "Poor Mom—this must be awful for her!" and "How would I feel if my kids put *me* in a home?" may indicate that a family member is *overidentifying* with the care receiver's plight and *projecting* his or her private, personal worries into the situation.
- *Omnipotence.* There's one in every family…smarter, wiser, and more insightful than the rest of us. Cousin Bert couldn't attend the initial meetings, of course, but now he's here, and he's going to fix everything up for you. Don't fall for this ploy. Your plan might not be perfect, but it's agreed-upon and in place. Hold your ground when your know-it-all cousin stops by: Stick with your plan, and make adjustments later.
- *Denial.* "Mom seems fine today—she seems perfectly normal. Maybe things aren't as bad as we thought." Denial is a natural reaction to negative events—a last-ditch effort to avoid the inevitable. Denial is normal, but don't give in to it. If you do, you'll undo all your hard work and be back to square one when the next crisis occurs. And believe us—it will.

Common Care-Receiver Objections

Chances are, your loved one will be scared and angry when you raise the prospect of nursing home placement. Can you blame her? As we discussed in Chapter 1, most people think of nursing home placement as a horrible thing, and they'll do almost anything to avoid it and stay in their home. Put yourself in the care receiver's place. You'd probably respond the exact same way.

Here are the kinds of objections you're likely to hear at this point, along with some suggestions for dealing with them:

Excuses

- *I don't need help.* "I was just having a bad day." "I had the flu." The explanations are endless. To counter these, let your loved one know that your concerns didn't arise from a single incident, but from a sustained pattern of behavior. Use specific examples to illustrate your concerns. Be ready to show that you're not overreacting to a single event, but to a series of problems that indicate a clear need for help.

- *I can't leave the house.* Houses are like pets—they can withstand brief absences, but soon begin to deteriorate without daily care and attention. "I can't leave the house" might be an excuse, or it might be a genuine concern on the care receiver's part. Either way, it's something you'll have to deal with down the line, especially in a suburban or rural area. For now, reassure her that the house will be looked after while she's away—she has your word on it. (We discuss strategies for managing the care receiver's house in her absence in Chapter 6.)

- *Your brother needs me.* This might be true, but it doesn't change the fact that the care receiver now needs help as well. If your loved one has been the primary caregiver for an ailing spouse, or a handicapped sibling or child, you're facing an especially thorny predicament. You'll have to seek placement for two people instead of one, and they might not be eligible for the same setting (though most nursing homes will make an effort to accommodate married residents).

Guilt-tripping

- *You wouldn't do this if your father were alive.* This statement will tug at your heartstrings, but it is an easy objection to counter if you recognize what she's really saying. The implication, of course, is that you're taking advantage of a helpless person. Explain to your loved one that you're not trying to get away with something—you simply want her to have the best possible care. And point out that she is hardly helpless. The fact that she's fighting with you over this is proof of her feistiness.

- *I cared for my parents—why can't you?* This needs to be addressed tactfully but honestly. The truth is, unless your parent was a physician or nurse with a lot of help from others, your grandparents probably didn't get the best care possible. And unless you're a skilled health care provider who can afford to quit work, you aren't going to be able to give your parent adequate care either.

Point out the financial constraints here, and explain that this approach is not realistic given your current situation.

- *After all I've done for you....* The implication here is, it's payback time: She took care of you, now you do the same. Your best strategy is to reframe the situation so your parent can see things differently. You are paying her back—not by parenting her (as she did for you), but by doing whatever is needed to ensure that her needs will be met as fully as possible.

Threats

- *I'm getting a lawyer.* The easiest way to counter this is not to counter it at all. Instead, respond that she should get a lawyer if she feels that strongly about it. She'll probably drop the matter right there, but if she insists on pursuing it, try to steer her toward a reputable attorney experienced in elder law. Chances are, the attorney will back you up. If the attorney disagrees and thinks nursing home placement is not warranted, don't get angry. Ask her why, and listen carefully to her answer. She might be right.

- *I'm taking you out of the will.* This can be intimidating, because let's face it—who wants to be disinherited? It will take a lot of gumption to stick to your guns in the face of this threat, but if you can, do. Acknowledge your loved one's feelings, restate your concerns, and explain how your proposal would address her needs. And don't be afraid to guilt-trip her back: Tell her if that's what it takes, you're willing to give up your inheritance so she can get good care.

- *I'd rather die, and when I do, it'll be on your head.* If you're hearing this now, you've probably heard it (or something quite like it) before, in response to other situations. Perhaps it's your loved one's habitual response to not getting her way. In any case, do not allow her (or anyone else for that matter) to engage in this type of emotional blackmail. Tell your loved one that if this is how she really feels, you'll be glad to get her the mental health treatment she needs. If she persists in repeating the threat, do just that.

Recognizing and Accepting the Person's Fears

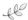

You must not give in to the care receiver's objections, but you should understand them. In part, these objections stem from an inaccurate view of what nursing homes are like, but in part they stem from some realistic fears and concerns. Growing old in a society like ours, where elderly people are discarded rather than valued, can be difficult. Being "put away" by those you trust makes it that much worse. When your loved one objects to nursing home care, here's what she's really afraid of:

- *Loss of status and self-esteem.* In most Western cultures, we define ourselves by what we do. When you imply that people can no longer function on their own, they begin to wonder whether they have any value anymore—to their family, friends, or society as a whole. Remember, too, that at some point your loved one is going to have to explain the situation to others. Having to tell his friends that he is being "put away" in a nursing home is, in a word, embarrassing.
- *Loss of freedom and autonomy.* We're used to running our own lives, calling our own shots, doing our own things. When we have to rely on others for help, some of that autonomy is taken from us. Dependency is scary—particularly when one must depend on one's children (who'll always be babies in their parents' eyes).
- *Loss of friends and social contacts.* Being in a nursing home makes it difficult to maintain friendships with those on the outside. The prospective nursing home resident may fear—quite reasonably—that she'll be abandoned by lifelong friends who can't (or won't) make the effort to visit. The care receiver may believe that nursing home placement will "disconnect" her from her familiar social world—a frightening prospect for anyone.

Developing a Partnership with the Care Receiver

Understanding the care receiver's fears and concerns will help you develop a partnership—a "working relationship" that is invaluable when difficult decisions must be made. Several strategies are useful here:

- *Reaffirm the value of the care receiver.* Don't assume the care re-

---

DRIVER'S ED

Obtaining a driver's license is one of our first tangible markers of adult responsibility. As time goes by, we tend to see driving not as a privilege but as a right. Driving is an integral part of independent living, particularly for people in areas that lack public transportation. No wonder most of us are reluctant to give it up.

When a person accustomed to going where she pleases must surrender her driver's license and rely on others to transport her, the loss is profound. The headaches for those who must take over driving duty are significant as well (which helps explain why people are often reluctant to insist that it's time for Mom or Dad to give up the car). Oftentimes we put off this difficult discussion until the inevitable happens: The older driver's slowed reaction time and diminished vision lead to a series of fender-benders, or even a serious accident. Then it's not simply a discussion; it's a crisis.

If your loved one is no longer driving safely, here are some options:

- Encourage them to take an over-55 defensive driving class. The material helps reinforce good driving habits in those whose last formal "Driver's Ed" took place decades ago. An added plus: Taking a defensive driving class reduces auto insurance rates in many states.
- Speak to your loved one's doctor about your concerns. He or she may recommend some formal vision and reaction-time tests and suggest appropriate intervention (for example, cataract removal to improve vision, or physical therapy to decrease reaction time).
- Contact your local Department of Motor Vehicles, and ask about policies and procedures for license restrictions. In most cases the care receiver's physician will need to be involved in this process, and attest in writing that the person can no longer drive safely.

ceiver understands your motivations. In fact, she may be assuming the worst—that you're just trying to "get rid of her." Tell her why you're doing this: Because you love her, you're concerned about her, and you want her to be safe, comfortable, and happy. You might need to provide this reassurance many times—perhaps every time the care receiver feels threatened or frightened—but that's OK. If it makes the person feel better, say it again.

- *Put the care receiver in charge.* To help the care receiver feel that she still has control, let her know that the family is her caregiving team, and she's the CEO. Her needs and desires are central to the decision-making process—they will never be ignored. She might not be able to have everything just the way she'd like it, but the primary goal of the team is to preserve her vision of the future—whatever it may be—in the context of current realities.

- *Clarify everyone's role.* Once you've put your loved one in charge of the operation, clarify everyone's role within the organization—who'll do what, who answers to whom, and so forth. Draw an organizational chart if you have to, with the care receiver at the top. Put everyone's name where it belongs on the chart, with their telephone number and e-mail address alongside. When something goes wrong, she'll know who to contact.

- *Put it in writing.* If the care receiver continues to express concerns about loss of freedom and autonomy, she might appreciate a written "contract" with the family, indicating who's responsible for what tasks (driving her to church, feeding the cat, etc.). Don't make promises you can't keep (even an informal contract may be legally binding), but everyone can benefit from a written agreement. Everyone (including the care receiver) should sign the contract, and everyone should get a copy.

When Your Loved One Is Determined to Disagree

Sometimes, despite your best efforts, the care receiver will hold her ground, and steadfastly refuse to consider nursing home care in any way, shape, or form. This can be frustrating, but if your loved one is not in immediate danger, you'll have to accept her decision. Keep the information you've collected, continue to investigate different options, and remind your loved one that you've made a commitment to help her obtain an appropriate level of care whenever she is ready to accept it.

If your loved one *is* in immediate danger, you must press forward despite her objections. You're doing the right thing, but be aware that some nasty arguments are likely to ensue. The family's best defense is to stick together, supporting each other in their decision. If the care receiver is genuinely unable to look after herself, and continues to resist a higher level of care, you might have to take action that could result in involuntary treatment.

In many areas, there are special crisis intervention services (usually called *geriatric evaluation services* or *geriatric assessment teams*) for elderly people who are resisting urgently needed care. Sponsored by local hospitals, mental health authorities, and agencies on aging, these teams of nurses, social workers, and mental health counselors are specially trained to assess older adults. At the re-

WHEN INDIVIDUAL RIGHTS CONFLICT WITH PUBLIC SAFETY

Balancing the rights of individuals with those of society can be tricky. Our democratic heritage is founded on each person's right to live life as he or she chooses. However, when the individual's freedom of choice puts others in danger, the greater good must prevail. Your loved one's desire to remain in her own apartment should be taken seriously, but if her confusion leads to a forgotten pot on the stove that creates a fire hazard, not only will she be harmed, but others may be as well.

When facing difficult decisions involving those we love, it's easy to underestimate the risk that a dangerous situation will occur. Don't. The costs are simply too great.

quest of family, friends, or others, the team will visit the home of an elderly person and assess the situation. Team members have the authority to bring the person to a hospital for more extensive evaluation and/or treatment, even if the person objects. If the person's competency is called into question as a result of these in-home and hospital assessments, legal procedures can be initiated to ensure that she will receive appropriate services.

The Concept of Competency

Competency is the formal, legal term that describes one's ability to function independently. If an individual is deemed legally incompetent, that person will be provided with a guardian or conservator, who will make decisions on his or her behalf. To be legally competent, a person must be able to:

- Obtain and apply needed information
- Reason in accordance with a set of values and beliefs
- Communicate the basis of his or her decisions to others

While the procedures vary from state to state, the process of having a person declared incompetent involves three basic steps:

- *Step 1: Initiating a hearing.* Someone, usually a family member, must go to court and formally question the person's ability to care for herself.
- *Step 2: The competency evaluation.* The individual who initiated the hearing requests that the person's competence be evaluated by a court-appointed representative. If the court agrees, the competency evaluation takes place, and the results of the evaluation are assessed by the court.
- *Step 3: Appointment of a guardian or conservator.* If the person is deemed incompetent, the court appoints someone—usually called a *guardian* or *conservator*—who assumes responsibility for making decisions on the person's behalf in those areas wherein they are incompetent. Guardians and conservators are monitored closely by the courts and must be prepared for audit or review at any time.

Keep in mind that under United States law, a person is considered competent until proven otherwise. Proof of incompetence must be substantial and must show that the person's current mental state constitutes a danger to self or others. To prevent people from having family members deemed incompetent unfairly (perhaps for personal benefit), evidence demonstrating incompetence must be reliable and unbiased. Thus, a judge in a competency hearing will often request that the individual be examined by lawyers, physicians, and psy-

WHEN STRUCTURE IS NEEDED: SOME ADDITIONAL OPTIONS

Sometimes people need a bit of extra help and structure, even though the situation is not serious enough to warrant nursing home placement. In these situations, there are several options:

- *Senior Centers.* Most communities have senior centers that provide lunch, an opportunity to socialize, and a variety of structured activities. Participants are expected to be in reasonably good health and able to get around with minimal assistance. Senior centers usually offer transportation to and from the building, and make regular trips to grocery stores, banks, and shopping malls. They may also offer day trips and at-cost entry to special events (like holiday concerts). Most centers are open during business hours on weekdays, but some are open round-the-clock (particularly those in cities with large senior populations).
- *Day Treatment Programs.* These are usually—but not always—housed in skilled nursing centers or hospitals. Day treatment staff include nurses, recreational therapists, and social workers. Some limited assistance with complex (but not basic) ADLs is available, including medication administration if needed. Participants are usually less independent than those at senior centers, and activities tend to focus on basic needs and interests (for example, exercise, current events discussion groups, cognitive stimulation, and socialization). Day treatment programs sometimes organize special events tailored to the interests of program participants, but the primary emphasis here is on maintaining participants' current level of functioning.
- *Partial Hospitalization Programs.* Usually housed in mental health centers, these are time-limited programs that provide medical and nursing supervision and a range of therapies to patients who have clearly defined needs and treatment goals. Admission to a partial hospitalization program must be initiated by a physician, and costs are often covered by Medicare and secondary insurance. Patients in partial hospitalization programs are generally at a lower level of functioning than those in day treatment programs. Like day treatment, partial hospitalization programs usually take place during business hours on weekdays, but some programs also have provisions for weekend or overnight coverage.

CAN COMPETENT DECISIONS STEM FROM CRAZY BELIEFS?

The answer is, it depends. It depends on how "crazy" the beliefs really are. If Mom won't use banks because the tellers are all Martians, this might well represent evidence of incompetence. However, if she keeps all her savings in cash because she thinks banks can't be trusted, that's her decision. If Dad won't see the doctor because he thinks the doctor's trying to poison him, this might be evidence of incompetence. However, if Dad's religious beliefs forbid him from entering heaven without all his parts, he has the right to refuse a leg amputation—no matter what the consequences.

chologists who have no interest in the outcome of the case before rendering a decision.

Remember, too, that competency isn't an all-or-nothing concept. A person can be incompetent in some areas and not others. It may be, for example, that a person can still carry out basic ADLs but has lost the ability to make sound financial decisions. Or the person may be able to communicate effectively but unable to manage her household. Thus, the parameters of guardianship and conservatorship vary according to the needs of the care receiver:

- *Guardianship can be partial or complete.* It can relate to some or all areas of the person's life.
- *Guardianship can be assigned to a single individual or to different people for different areas.* Sometimes one person makes decisions about health care, while another makes decisions about finances or living arrangements.
- *Guardianship can be assigned to people other than family members.* While family members are usually appointed as conservators or guardians, in some cases these duties are delegated to other people who, in the eyes of the court, can make sound, objective decisions in the best interests of the individual (for example, bank trustees).

As with most legal matters, competency arrangements are never written in stone. People can regain competency when their health status improves, and guardianships can be revoked or altered as circumstances change. Altering or re-voking guardianship or conservatorship is a legal process that follows well-defined state and federal laws. You'll need an experienced elder law attorney to manage this process properly.

If You're in Charge

If you're the sole guardian or conservator for decision-making about your loved one's care, you have the final word. Others may disagree, but they cannot alter your decisions unless they choose to challenge you legally—a complicated and costly process. If you're in charge, and you think nursing home placement is warranted, you can make it happen—even if the care receiver objects.

The situation differs if you're sharing responsibility with others. In this case, you all have a voice and the authority to challenge each another's decisions. Not surprisingly, conflict is common when power is shared. When it gets out of hand it can result in sheer chaos (and some nasty legal battles as well). For these reasons, sole guardianship or conservatorship is usually preferable to shared guardianship or conservatorship.

If you share decision-making responsibility with others, you must find some way to cooperate and work together as a team. The guardians or conservators should:

- Meet regularly to review decisions, and determine whether those decisions are still working well.
- Document what takes place during meetings—keep written minutes at the very least, tape recordings if necessary.
- Learn to argue constructively and tolerate disagreement. (Use the family meeting strategies we discussed earlier in this chapter.)
- Remind yourselves frequently why you're there: To meet your loved one's needs, not your own. (It sounds simple, but it's easy to forget.)
- Get used to settling on compromise solutions: This is not a good arena to play out sibling rivalries, and nobody "wins" if your loved one's care is compromised.

5

Choosing the Right Placement Setting: Thinking Clearly in the Midst of Chaos

This place is huge! The Admissions Office is in the main building, almost a half-mile from the edge of the campus. Along the way there are rows of freestanding homes and townhouses. The lawns are perfect, fringed with lilacs—here and there a rose trellis or grape arbor. It seems strangely peaceful, and then I realize why: There are no children playing in the yards. All you hear is the whoosh of sprinklers and the tinkle of wind chimes.

Finally, I enter the parking lot. There's a visitor's area off to the side, past the long row of blue-painted handicapped spots. As I approach the building, I see a group of people in wheelchairs, talking as they watch the cars come and go. A middle-aged woman in white sits with them, gesturing broadly as she speaks. They pause as I pass. One woman waves, several nod; a man calls out, "Good morning!"

Two automatic doors open as I enter. The lobby looks like the reception area of a large hotel. Chairs are clustered near floor-to-ceiling windows that look out on flowered courtyards. A dozen older folks are lounging and chatting, checking purses and totebags, and I gather they're waiting for a bus to go to town. A few have canes, and many wear hearing aids; all are neatly dressed for the trip. I check in with the receptionist, then sit on a nearby couch. Over the music in the waiting area I hear the sound of the intercom—paging staff members, announcing meeting times, giving highlights of the daily news.

The Admissions Director doesn't seem surprised when I tell her this place doesn't look like I'd expected. Her office is equipped with a large desk and racks filled with forms and pamphlets. A large-print "Residents' Bill of Rights" takes up much of one wall, near framed pictures of older people eating, walking, and dancing. The Admission Director's desk is busy—piled high with folders, newsletters, cards, and notes.

She suggests we take a tour while she tells me about the facility. Half an hour later, I wish I'd worn sneakers. The main dining room is bright and airy, filled with tables for four and six, all set with place-cards. The physical therapy suite looks like a professional gym, with weights, parallel bars, and mats. Behind a glass wall there's a pool, with a whirlpool nearby. Then we're on to the craft shop, with work benches and project-strewn tables, and past that the beauty shop, which is filled with clients. Along the way we pass two—no, three— television lounges with large-screen, closed-caption sets. Finally, we make our way down a hallway to the chapel, which is simple but cheerful. In the front pew a couple sits quietly, with books held open in their laps. The Admissions Director smiles at me, puts a finger to her lips. We close the door softly and head back to her office.

Not what you'd expect a nursing home to look like, is it? Many people are pleas-antly surprised when they visit a long-term care facility for the first time. Many look more like resort hotels than hospitals—hardly the depressing "warehouse" that we picture when we think of a nursing home.

Appearances aside, nursing homes vary tremendously with respect to qual-ity, cost, and other important factors. In this chapter, we discuss strategies for choosing the right setting when long-term care is needed.

Varieties of Placement Settings

In many cases, your loved one's medical needs will dictate the level of care he or she required, but sometimes a person's needs are less clear-cut, and choices must be made. Oftentimes people move through a series of out-of-home care options, rather than going straight from their home to the nursing home. Here are key features of different living and treatment settings for seniors.

Senior communities

Senior communities (also called *congregate housing*) are private communities for independent older people who prefer neighbors of their own age. Eligibility is based on age and functional level, though criteria vary from community to community. Rent includes maintenance and use of common areas; other expenses (like utilities) are paid for by the resident. Senior communities are usually located near public transportation, shopping districts, and medical centers. Funding is out-of-pocket, though government subsidies are sometimes available for low-income seniors.

Most senior communities were constructed with accessibility in mind. Doorways and walkways are wheelchair-accessible, bathrooms are designed with grab bars and "roll-in" showers, doors have easy-open handles. Some senior communities also provide a "medic-alert" system to summon help quickly in emergencies. Senior communities are best suited to high-functioning elders, and unless the senior community is part of a "continuing care community" (described later in this chapter), the resident may have to leave if he or she develops significant direct care needs.

Group homes

These are supervised households that include elderly and disabled residents whose primary needs are for companionship and housekeeping services. Funding is out-of-pocket and usually includes room, board, laundry, and some transportation. Staff are present on a twenty-four-hour basis. Assistance is available for basic medical needs (such as monitoring blood pressure) and occasionally for bathing and dressing as well. Most group homes can accommodate wheelchair-bound residents, but few are equipped to deal with more significant mobility limitations, incontinence, or serious medical conditions.

Most require that the resident find housing elsewhere if she develops any of these problems.

Assisted living facilities

Assisted living facilities are designed for people who need help with complex ADLs on a daily basis. They provide private or semiprivate rooms with attached baths in buildings with communal dining and living areas. Some assisted living facilities are freestanding, but many are housed on the grounds of nursing centers or continuing care communities. Funding is out-of-pocket (although some long-term-care insurance policies pay a percentage of the costs), and the basic fee usually covers room, board, laundry, and transportation. Most assisted living facilities offer social programming, but this can vary quite a bit depending on the size of the facility and the resident mix.

Staff are available around the clock to provide help with bathing, dressing, and basic medical needs (such as blood glucose monitoring). Some facilities offer incontinence care, and most will assist residents with medication administration if state law permits. (This varies from state to state—ask ahead of time.) Assisted living facilities do not provide skilled nursing care, so the resident must move to a facility that provides a higher level of care if he develops serious medical problems.

"AGING IN PLACE": AN ALTERNATIVE TO ASSISTED LIVING

It makes sense when you think about it: Seniors who need some assistance with living—but don't need formal "assisted living"—band together to form cooperatives designed to provide the extra help that will allow them to live at home. These "Aging in Place" communities are appearing in every region of the country, and they all work pretty much the same way. Groups of seniors pool their resources, contributing to a fund that is used to provide services like minor home repairs, meal preparation, yard care, computer tech support, check-in calls, and transportation to and from appointments. Volunteers from within the group provide some services; others are provided by local professionals at discounted rates. Annual fees to join an Aging in Place group in 2008 ranged from $500 to $900 per household. For information regarding Aging in Place philosophy and programs, contact the Center of Aging in Place Support at 914-315-6491 (www.aipsupport.org).

Skilled care facilities

As the name implies, skilled care facilities offer extensive nursing services for those with significant medical needs. Different levels of service are available, depending on the complexity of the resident's care needs. Admission must be initiated by the person's physician, and services deemed "medically necessary" are usually covered, at least in part, by Medicare, Medicaid, or other insurance. Skilled care facilities fall into two general categories: *rehab care* and *special care*.

- *Rehab care.* Usually located in hospitals or nursing homes, rehab care programs (sometimes called "Level 1," acute care, or transitional care) provide intensive medical care for patients who are expected to regain functional capacity and return home within a relatively short time. The typical patient in such a program was first admitted to a hospital for surgery, or for treatment of an injury or acute illness, and now requires a period of rehabilitation to facilitate recovery. Medicare usually covers the majority of costs for room and board, nursing care, and physician-prescribed therapies during the first one hundred days, as long as the patient continues to improve and shows adequate motivation to participate in treatment.

- *Special care.* There are two types of special care units. Some offer specialized care for patients with specific medical needs (for example, a ventilator for breathing, a feeding tube to provide nourishment). These units are often identified by the type of service they provide (for example, "vent units" or "tube units"), or they may simply be referred to as "Level 2" care. Other special care units are set up to deal with behavioral problems that stem from dementia (such as aggressiveness or wandering). These units are usually "secure," have high staff-to-patient ratios, and provide comprehensive programming for confused, disoriented residents.

Long-term care

Long-term-care settings are what most of us think of when we picture a nursing home. These are long-term living options for people deemed unlikely to return to independent living. Residents will occasionally show tremendous improvement in long-term care, but this rarely occurs in cases of Alzheimer's disease or other forms of dementia. The patients who improve most are usually those recovering from injury or surgery—people in the midst of rehab, but who haven't recovered within the allowed time limits (at which point insurance guidelines dictate that further treatment must take place in a long-term-care facility).

Long-term care includes nursing supervision, but it is primarily custodial ("maintenance") care rather than skilled care. Services are aimed at keeping the person safe and healthy, but not at improving his condition. Because of this, Medicare rarely covers the cost of long-term care (though Medicaid will cover these costs for eligible residents). Long-term-care costs are sometimes covered by long-term-care insurance policies, though the specifics vary from policy to policy; it's best to check on this ahead of time.

Continuing Care Communities

Continuing care communities (also called *step care* or *progressive care* communities) offer a full range of options, from independent living through special care. In most cases, residents must be independent on admission, but once admitted they become eligible for the entire spectrum of services. Private homes in continuing care communities are not relinquished until there is no possibility of return to independent living, which provides tremendous security for the resident. The downside of this policy is that vacancies in continuing care communities tend to be rare, since turnover is slow. A house or apartment may remain empty for weeks—even months—while its occupant is receiving treatment in another part of the facility.

As you might guess, security like this doesn't come cheap. Initial out-of-pocket entry fees range from $50,000 to $400,000 or more. Most or all of this entry fee is nonrefundable, which makes moving into a continuing care community a bit of a gamble: If the resident dies soon after admission, the cost per day could turn out to be astronomical. (That rarely happens, though—the typical length of stay is about five years.)

In addition to entry fees, residents pay for services they use (electric, telephone, etc.), and monthly maintenance fees, which increase over time. Because most continuing care communities offer a wide range of care options, it is unlikely that a resident's needs will exceed what the facility can provide. However, if for some reason the resident requires a lengthy off-grounds stay, maintenance and rental/mortgage fees must still be paid (a serious financial strain for fixed-income residents).

Entry into a continuing care community involves some unusual financial arrangements. Because entry fees are held in escrow accounts, they do not count as personal assets (which can speed the resident's Medicaid eligibility). Another financial quirk involves property ownership: In those cases where the property is purchased by the resident, there are strict rules regarding resale and refinancing, so the community controls the property after the resident dies.

Most facilities have stringent rules regarding noise, pets, vehicles, and exterior decorations. Guests are monitored closely, and some facilities forbid children or teenagers from staying overnight. Most communities allow only married couples or blood relatives to share a home, and many exclude couples with nontraditional lifestyles. On the other hand, some communities are now targeting the needs of gay and lesbian elders and other seniors with nontraditional living situations.

HOUSING OPTIONS: THE BOTTOM LINE

Option	Who is it for?	What does it cost? Who pays for it?	What are its advantages?
Senior Communities	Independent seniors	$1,500 to $2,000 per month or more; limited Medicaid funding for low-income seniors	A homelike setting with extra services
Group Homes	People who need help with complex ADLs	$1,200-$2,000 per month; long-term care insurance may cover part of cost (limited Medicaid funding for low-income seniors)	Homelike (group) setting with twenty-four-hour emergency coverage

Option	Who is it for?	What does it cost? Who pays for it?	What are its advantages?
Assisted Living Facilities	People who need help with basic and complex ADLs	$2,000+ per month; sometimes covered by long-term-care insurance	High level of care with some independence
Skilled Care Facilities	People with significant short-term care needs	$3,000-$4,000 per month (more for rehab or special care); may be covered in part by Medicare, Medicaid, and private insurance	Twenty-four-hour access to skilled nursing and medical care
Long-Term Care	People unlikely to resume independent living	$60,000 per year and up; covered by Medicaid and long-term-care insurance	Ongoing custodial care and supervision
Continuing Care	Independent people who want access to higher levels of care, if needed	$1,500 to $5,000 per month or more, plus a substantial entry fee; paid for out-of-pocket	Guaranteed care for future health problems

Obtaining Information About a Specific Setting

A decade ago, finding a good nursing home could be difficult. Today, new ones are opening everywhere—good news for the consumer, because choice creates competition, and competition helps control prices. As you explore placement options, you'll be courted aggressively offered tours, brochures, even videos.

MARKETING TECHNIQUES TO WATCH FOR

Most nursing home marketing directors are trustworthy, but some unscrupulous people might try to sell you a service more costly than you need. Three "hard sell" approaches to watch for:

- *The Foot-in-the-Door Technique.* This involves getting you to agree to a modest request, then upping the ante and asking you to purchase something larger. If a marketing director gets you to agree to a care program or rooming arrangement with modest costs, then starts adding in "hidden" features that increase the price substantially, you are being manipulated via the foot-in-the-door technique. Demand to hear the "bottom-line" cost, with everything included.
- *The Door-in-the-Face Technique.* When this technique is used, the marketing person makes a large request, which you are expected to turn down, then follows it up with a smaller request, to which you agree. You might not think this strategy would work, but it does: Studies show that once we turn down a large request, we are actually more likely to agree to a smaller request (perhaps out of guilt, or because the smaller request seems cheap by comparison). We may even agree to a smaller request we had no intention of purchasing when the door-in-the-face strategy is used.
- *The Reciprocity Strategy.* This involves making you feel indebted (usually by giving you something "free"). You are then more likely to agree to the gift giver's requests, because you feel that you owe him something in return for the things you received. Free videos or long-term-care planning guides, free cookies and soft drinks—all may be telltale signs of the reciprocity strategy at work.

Keep in mind that marketing materials are just that: advertisements designed to sell you a product. As with any purchase, you must move beyond the hype to make a fully informed decision.

As you explore placement options, you should do four things: *get technical ratings, talk to administrators, talk to residents and their families,* and *inspect the facility.* On page 237, we provide a Nursing Home Comparison Checklist to take with you when you visit different facilities, so you can be sure you cover everything. Here's how to go about getting the information you need:

Getting technical ratings

Certified nursing facilities are subject to regular inspection by federal and state agencies, and the results of these surveys must be made available to anyone who asks. As you'll see, these inspections are extremely thorough, and include details that might seem trivial (like water temperature), but that have important implications for residents. (Too-hot water leads to scalding accidents.) When a facility doesn't meet some standard, it must implement a "plan of correction," which is also reviewed by the appropriate agencies. Deficiencies can result in hefty fines—up to $10,000 per violation per day.

Ask to see each facility's most recent survey findings and plans of correction, and read them carefully. Ask questions about deficiencies and the remedies implemented. Don't expect a facility to be perfect—almost every facility has at least a few minor problems. Rather than looking for a problem-free place, look for a place that tackles problems effectively.

Here are some issues to focus on as you examine these ratings:

- *Safety issues* (number of falls, injuries, deaths)
- *Quality of care issues* (frequency of medication errors, wounds, hygiene violations)
- *Staffing patterns* (staff credentials, appropriateness of services)
- *Quality of life issues* (freedom from unnecessary restraints and restrictions, resident satisfaction ratings)

Talking to administrators

The first person you'll meet at each facility will probably be a member of the admissions or marketing staff. That person can provide written materials, financial information, and other basics. They'll usually give you a tour of the grounds as well and introduce you to staff members you encounter along the way.

If possible, try to meet the facility's Chief Administrator and Director of Nursing during your visit. In most settings, the Chief Administrator is in charge of all business aspects of the operation; the Director of Nursing oversees day-to-day hands-on care. These two people can answer most of your questions, and their demeanor will give you a feel for the tone of the facility.

If you have the opportunity to speak with members of the direct care staff during your tour, you'll get an even better sense of how the place runs. If you can't speak with direct care staff during your tour, try to observe how they interact with the residents. Do they seem friendly? Relaxed? Harried? Crabby? Would you want them working with your mother?

Here are key questions to ask nursing home administrators:

- How did you do on your last survey?
- How many residents live here now, and how does that compare to the facility's actual capacity?
- What's the average length of stay?
- Where do residents go when they leave the facility?
- How many direct care staff are employed here?
- What's the staff-to-patient ratio on each shift?
- How do you recruit and retain good staff?
- What are your staff turnover patterns?
- What services are provided by outside contractors and independent providers?
- Where could the facility improve?
- What steps are you taking to accomplish this?

Talking to residents and their families

Nobody knows a place better than the people who live there. Because residents and their families have certain privacy rights, you will rarely be introduced to them during your tour. But you may find that if you take the initiative, many residents and their families are happy to offer their opinions. Admissions staff might also provide you with contact information for current and former residents who have agreed to share their experiences. (Of course, the facility is going to steer you toward those clients who had positive experiences, so you need to keep this in mind as you assess what you hear.)

Here are key questions to ask residents and their families:

- How long have you lived here?
- Have there been many changes since you arrived?
- What do you like most about this place?
- What would you change about this place, if you could?
- Are your needs met promptly?
- Do staff members address problems appropriately?

- Do staff members treat you with respect?
- Are you satisfied with the staff?
- Do you have enough to do? (Are you ever bored?)
- How's the food?

BEWARE THE ANCIENT MARINER

Life in a nursing home can be frustrating, and on occasion an angry resident will waylay touring visitors at the front door to vent grievances (sometimes in excruciating detail). While this might give you pause, keep in mind that a good facility will encourage freedom of speech rather than attempting to suppress complaints; some degree of grumbling among the residents is actually a healthy sign.

So how can you separate genuine problems from random complaints? Two ways. First, when chatting with residents about their experiences, try to assess the plausibility of their criticisms. "The food here is foul!" could mean exactly that, but it could also reflect the absence of that resident's favorite dish, or the occasional cup of cold coffee. Second, listen for patterns, common themes that come up again and again among different residents. These are the issues to take seriously, and the ones that can help you decide whether a particular facility should be avoided.

Inspecting the Facility

As was true in selecting a home-care worker (Chapter 3), not all the information you need to evaluate a nursing home can be obtained by asking questions. You also need to inspect the facility yourself, using your powers of observation to make your own assessments in key areas.

The physical setting

Several characteristics distinguish a well-run nursing home from one that is poorly run:

- *Cleanliness.* Places that house sick and incontinent people generate some pretty noxious odors, but a good facility knows how to handle this. It should have adequate ventilation and a neutral or pleasant smell. This is not to suggest that some spots won't be a bit whiffy—soiled laundry carts are soiled laundry carts. However, the overall air quality should be comparable to that in your own home. Floors and furniture should be clean and stain-free. Linens and laundry should look reasonably fresh.

- *Accessibility.* To meet the needs of disabled residents, doors should be equipped with push bars or automatic swing mechanisms. Entrances and hallways should be wide enough to accommodate wheelchairs and walkers. If there are multiple floors, elevators should be clearly marked. Public rooms should be labeled with easy-to-decipher symbols. If cabinets aren't reachable from wheelchairs, "grabbers" should be available. Some of the lounge chairs should be low, with sturdy arms for easy access. Lights should be bright so that people with limited vision can read without difficulty. Telephones should be equipped with amplifiers; televisions in common areas should have headphones nearby.

- *Upkeep.* Care facilities are high-traffic places and require a lot of maintenance. Try to focus on those features that affect health and safety, rather than decor. (Faded wallpaper isn't a health hazard; a torn carpet is.) Older fixtures or furniture might not be

---

NURSING HOMES NEAR AND FAR

Location is an important—but neglected—factor in nursing home choice. The facility should be close enough to allow convenient access for family members and others who will be involved in the resident's life. If the nursing home is located in the suburbs, or in a rural area, remember that at some point weather will be an issue. If you're checking out the facility in July, try to picture what driving there during a January snowstorm would be like. If the nursing home is at the end of a mile-long single-lane road, it will be difficult to reach when the weather's bad.

pretty, but sometimes these things help residents feel at home. Be on the lookout for slippery floors and other warning signs of a poorly kept facility.

The milieu

Evaluating the physical setting is relatively straightforward. Assessing the milieu—the interpersonal environment—is trickier. Here's what to look for:

- *Roommate considerations.* In many nursing homes, private rooms are hard to come by (and they cost substantially more than shared space). Semiprivate rooms generally consist of a bedroom and bathroom (without shower or tub) shared by two to four people. Efforts are made to group compatible residents, but roommate conflicts remain one of the most common problems in nursing homes. Find out how roommates are chosen, how disputes are addressed, and what options residents have if problems prove insurmountable.
- *Resident mix.* Care facilities deal with people whose health is constantly changing. At some point, confused and disori-

---

WHAT TO EXPECT FROM OTHER NURSING HOME RESIDENTS

Most of the people you'll encounter during a nursing home tour will be calmly going about their business—reading, visiting, watching TV, chatting on the phone. However, if you've never been in a nursing home, you might not be prepared for some of the behaviors you encounter, particularly on special care units for demented residents. People may scream, moan, curse for no reason, talk incessantly, ask impolite questions, and make inappropriate remarks. Some may attempt to remove their clothes, or expose themselves. Others may be wet or soiled. The sights, sounds, and smells of these units can be extremely upsetting to first-time visitors. Keep in mind, these people are here for a reason: They had needs that exceeded their loved ones' abilities to care for them. And remember—you're in *their* home, which is designed to keep them safe and comfortable, not to shield you from the unpleasant aspects of their illness.

ented residents may be mixed in with alert and oriented folks. Many residents cope well with this if it's short-lived, but others are very uncomfortable in the presence of demented or agitated neighbors. Find out how the facility handles this situation. Are there special, secure areas for demented residents? Confused residents? Residents who wander, moan, steal, or scream?

The intangibles

Intangibles have to do with how a place *feels*—they are personal judgments that may be difficult to quantify. Nonetheless, intangibles can make a tremendous difference in the life of a resident. Begin by asking yourself two questions:

- *Does it seem friendly?* Some settings are spotless but impersonal. Others are a little worn around the edges but cozy and homey. Little things, like decorations and personal touches, can tell you a lot about how the staff feel about residents (and vice versa). Does this seem like a friendly, welcoming place?
- *Would I want to live there?* Well, that's not really a fair question: Of course not—it's a nursing home! Still, try to imagine yourself in your loved one's place, and ask yourself: Could I live here if I had to? How does it compare to others I've seen? What would I like about living here? What would drive me nuts?

Funding: Who Pays for What?

With good advance planning, out-of-pocket health care costs for an ill or aging loved one can be quite manageable. Without advance planning, the cost of care can wipe out a lifetime's worth of savings in a matter of weeks or months. There are several primary funding sources for long-term care.

Medicare

Medicare is a form of insurance designed to defray some out-of-pocket medical costs of elderly and disabled people. Medicare comes in four parts. Part A (which is funded by the taxes paid to FICA during a person's working years)

OTHER NURSING HOME "INTANGIBLES"

As you compare nursing homes, don't forget about these other "intangibles"—features of the facility that can be important down the line:

- *Size matters.* Nursing homes vary quite a bit in size, from intimate places that house a few dozen residents to large facilities with hundreds of patients. Both types of nursing homes have their own advantages. (Smaller facilities provide more personal attention; larger ones offer a broader range of services.) Consider ahead of time whether a small or large facility would be better for your loved one.
- *The religion question.* Some (but not all) nursing homes are closely affiliated with a particular religious group. Oftentimes this affiliation is apparent from the facility's name or its written materials. If religious affiliation is important to you or your loved one, ask about this up front.
- *Balancing the books.* The eldercare market is expanding rapidly, and many nursing homes have recently been taken over by large corporations. (Oftentimes these are the same corporations that run hotel chains.) Ask whether this is the case for each nursing home you visit, and don't be shy about requesting copies of each corporation's most recent annual report. Any financially sound company will be happy to provide this information.

covers certain hospital costs and is available to anyone over age sixty-five. Part B (which is available for an additional fee, whether or not the person has Part A coverage) covers aspects of outpatient care. Part C (also known as *Medicare Advantage Plan*) is available through Medicare-approved private insurance companies, and combines Medicare Parts A and B (it sometimes includes prescription drug coverage as well, depending upon the plan one chooses). Part D (which includes a variety of plans and varying levels of coverage and co-payment) covers prescription drug costs.

Medicare Parts C and D involve a range of options, and choices in both areas can be tricky. It may be worthwhile to check with a Certified Financial Planner before deciding whether to purchase Medicare Part C, and with the care receiver's physician before deciding which Medicare Part D plan to enroll in.

PURPLE HAZE: THE INS AND OUTS OF MEDICARE PART D

Medicare Part D is designed to cover the ever-increasing costs of prescription drugs for seniors—and it does, sort of. But when you look at the specifics, you might wonder what was going on in the minds of those who designed the plan. Consider...

Most Medicare Part D plans involve a monthly premium, an annual deductible, and a co-payment for each prescription. You always pay the monthly premium, plus 100 percent of your drug costs until you reach the deductible, which can range up to $250 or more, depending on the plan. Once you reach the deductible, you pay a certain percentage of your medication costs (depending on the plan) until you reach a threshold ($2,400 in 2007). You then begin paying 100 percent of your prescription costs again until you reach a second threshold, the "ceiling" amount ($3,850 in 2007). At this point Medicare picks up the entire cost for all additional prescription drugs that year.

Confused yet? Wait. Just to make it more interesting, drugs are classified into "formularies"—lists of medications that vary from plan to plan. If a drug prescribed by your doctor is not on the list, it won't be covered. There are also coverage "tiers," so even within a given formulary, some drugs are covered at nearly 100 percent, while others require the consumer to pay a higher percentage of the cost. All formularies include drugs needed for treatment of common medical conditions (e.g., diabetes, hypertension), but none cover everything. If your plan doesn't include most drugs in your medication regimen, you can change plans once a year, but some restrictions apply.

Medicare Part A will fund a portion of the costs for up to one hundred days of care in a certified skilled nursing facility. Medicare Part A coverage includes semiprivate room fees, meals, skilled nursing care, rehabilitation services (such as physical and speech therapies), medications, medical supplies, and medical equipment. The amount of coverage varies over time, as follows:

- *Days 1-20.* Generally, Medicare covers all costs during this period, except for the patient's annual deductible.
- *Days 21-100.* Medicare pays all but the designated co-insurance amount. The patient pays the co-insurance amount ($128.00 per day in 2008) out-of-pocket or through private secondary insurance.

• *After day 100.* From here on out, the patient pays the bills. Most secondary insurance policies will not cover co-insurance costs at this point (though some long-term-care policies do cover these costs—ask before you buy).

As you can see, today's Medicare system provides incentives for getting well quickly. In addition, benefits may be stopped at any time within the one-

---

SERVICES AND GOODS NOT COVERED BY MEDICARE

Knowing what Medicare *doesn't* cover is important too. Goods and services not covered by Medicare include:

• Custodial care
• Private rooms (unless medically necessary, as in cases of quarantine)
• Private duty nurses
• Any service provided by a noncertified facility
• Anything not considered medically necessary
• Telephones and televisions in the patient's room

THE ALZHEIMER'S-MEDICARE CATCH-22

Alzheimer's disease and the other forms of dementia present unique funding problems for care receivers and their families. The Alzheimer's patient may be quite healthy physically and therefore need little or no "skilled" care (making him or her Medicare-ineligible). At the same time, the person may be incapable of living safely without intensive, round-the-clock supervision. As you can imagine, this creates a real dilemma for caregivers. (The situation is a bit better for Medicaid recipients, because Medicaid covers the base costs of nursing home care—though not the cost of increased staffing and supervision.)

hundred-day period if the patient does not show adequate improvement. Worst of all from the patient's perspective, Medicare may deny payments retroactively: they can refuse to pay for services already delivered if they decide that the patient was ineligible for any reason. If this happens, the patient is responsible for services rendered but denied. And a verbal promise from a Medicare representative won't carry any weight when a retroactive denial occurs (though you can always appeal the decision).

As with any insurance policy, Medicare benefits are not paid automatically just because the patient is enrolled. To be eligible for reimbursement in a skilled nursing facility, the patient must meet two criteria:

- The patient must have been treated in a hospital for the illness in question for at least three consecutive days within thirty days of receiving skilled nursing care.
- The patient's physician must declare that treatment of the covered medical problem is medically necessary and that the person requires care on a daily basis.

As you can imagine, many medical conditions do not meet these criteria, and in these situations paying for treatment can become a complicated matter. There are also numerous exclusions for specific goods and services under Medicare Part A. The bottom line: Contrary to popular belief, Medicare pays only a small portion of the costs of nursing home care.

Medicaid

Medicaid is health insurance paid for by federal and state funds, to help cover medical costs for those in financial need. Medicaid pays the entire cost of basic nursing home care (no frills), along with dental work and prescription medications. Over the years, Medicaid has become a primary funding source for long-term care. (It now pays the bills for nearly 50 percent of all nursing home residents.) Because Medicaid reimbursement rates are set by the state—not the nursing home—Medicaid almost always pays for services at a lower rate than other insurance sources. Thus, facilities and service providers make less money on Medicaid patients, and many facilities no longer accept them. There are, however, two exceptions to this guideline:

- If a current resident becomes Medicaid-eligible, most nursing

MEDICARE AND MEDICAID CONTACT INFORMATION

A great deal of information can be found on the federal government's Medicare web site (www.medicare.gov), or by calling 800-633-4227. Medicaid information is a bit harder to obtain, because Medicaid funds are channeled through individual states. Your best bet is to look in the *Human Services* section of your phone book, contact the Centers for Medicare and Medicaid Services, and locate the contact information for your state.

homes will continue to work with them.
- If a facility accepts Medicaid, it is illegal for them to discharge Medicaid patients to make room for higher-paying patients.

Medicaid eligibility requirements vary from state to state, but in general, a person must have minimal income (usually less than $15,000 per year) and virtually no savings or financial resources that could be used to cover health care costs (in most states, less than $60,000 in total assets). In most states, excluded assets include the home (as long as at least one spouse is living in it), one vehicle, one wedding ring, one engagement ring, a life insurance policy not to exceed $1,500 face value, a burial plot, and a prepaid funeral plan.

Not surprisingly, many people have looked for ways to become Medicaid-eligible without first spending all their hard-earned resources on late-life health care. In the past, many patients got around this requirement by shifting assets into loved ones' names before receiving treatment, thereby creating the appearance of being destitute. These practices weren't limited to middle-income folks, either: Many wealthy people used these strategies to shelter large sums of money for their heirs, while using taxpayers' funds to pay their long-term-care bills.

Changes in Medicaid regulations have made many of these practices illegal, and there are harsh penalties—including jail terms—for those who cheat the system. Regulations known as "lookback rules" now specify exactly how long one must have had limited income and assets before becoming Medicaid-eligible. Thus:

- States may go back five years to determine whether a potential Medicaid-recipient's assets were transferred appropriately, so early planning is key.
- In determining Medicaid eligibility, the person's financial records will be scrutinized carefully. Omissions—intentional or otherwise—may be considered fraud, a very serious matter.
- If funds are transferred to another person via a trust, it must be an irrevocable trust, so funds cannot be transferred back to the Medicaid-recipient. (We discuss the basics of trusts and other financial matters in Chapter 6.)

THE TEN STANDARD MEDIGAP PLANS

Basic Benefits (which are covered by all ten plans) include: (1) Medicare Part A coinsurance costs, plus coverage for 365 days after Medicare benefits end; (2) Part B coinsurance costs; and (3) three pints of blood per year. Many of the covered services have yearly limits, exclusions, and deductible amounts, however. (These are described in each plan's written literature.)

Coverage:	A	B	C	D	E	F	G	H	I	J
Basic Benefits	X	X	X	X	X	X	X	X	X	X
Part A Deductible		X	X	X	X	X	X	X	X	X
Foreign Travel Emergency			X	X	X	X	X	X	X	X
Skilled Nursing Coinsurance			X	X	X	X	X	X	X	X
Part B Excess Charges						X	X		X	X
Part B Deductible			X		X					X
At-home Recovery Costs				X			X		X	X
Prescription Drugs								X	X	X
Preventive Care					X					X

Medigap insurance

Medicare Supplement Insurance (commonly called *Medigap* insurance) is privately funded health care coverage intended to pay some of the costs not covered by Medicare. Medigap policies are "guaranteed renewable"—your insurer cannot refuse to renew your policy as long as you pay your premiums on time and were truthful when you first applied for coverage.

There are ten standard Medigap policies (Plans "A" through "J"), which range from basic coverage through fairly comprehensive service. Efforts have been made to make the plans uniform across states and insurers, but some loopholes remain. For example, some states don't offer every Medigap option, and insurers are permitted to add extra benefits, thereby increasing costs. Most Medigap plans cover the deductible for Medicare Part A, co-insurance for hospital and skilled nursing care, and some outpatient costs. The more elaborate plans also cover some of the costs of prescription drugs, emergency care while abroad, preventive care, and in-home care.

Medicare SELECT plans are essentially Medigap policies sold by HMOs, which designate the specific doctors and hospitals you must use in order to get full coverage. Medicare still pays its share of approved charges, but like any HMO, the SELECT plan may not cover services rendered by out-of-network providers.

Secondary insurance

Some employers and professional organizations allow you to maintain existing group health coverage postretirement. You can also purchase health insurance privately (though costs can be prohibitive, and many policies exclude pre-existing conditions). Precisely what is covered by secondary insurance can vary quite a bit across policies, but generally speaking, it's getting increasingly selective every year: More and more services are being excluded or made difficult to access, and larger percentages of the costs are being shifted to the consumer through co-pays and deductibles. For some people, secondary insurance is an excellent safety net, but keep in mind that most secondary insurance policies do not cover long-term-care costs.

The rules that govern secondary policies differ from those for Medicare and Medigap. Determining who covers what when you have all three policies can be tricky (and spousal benefits are particularly difficult to decipher). Read your policies carefully, and consider getting advice from an insurance counselor familiar with the rules for your state. The consultation won't be free, but it can go a long way toward helping you understand exactly what is covered by each policy.

Long-term-care insurance

Long-term-care insurance is a relative newcomer to the insurance scene. It is designed to defray the costs of long-term custodial care for people unlikely to qualify for Medicaid. Long-term-care policies pay for a substantial portion of the costs of custodial care, and some newer policies are quite flexible—benefits may be used in a variety of treatment settings or even at home. According to year 2007 industry standards, long-term-care policies are best suited to those whose "non-excludable" assets are in excess of $200,000 and whose annual income is $30,000 or more. Most policies pay a fixed dollar amount toward each level of care, with more intensive care being reimbursed at a higher rate. There are often upper age limits and exclusions for pre-existing conditions.

Long-term-care insurance benefits are usually triggered by deterioration in ADLs, as determined by one's primary physician. This can be tricky, though—some policies will pay for services only if you need help with three or more ADLs. (Deterioration in two areas is not enough.) And some policies pay benefits only when the recipient is *physically* incapable of performing these tasks—if ADL deterioration stems from cognitive decline, the insurer won't pay. If possible, look for a policy that:

- Allows the holder to receive benefits when they need help with only one or two ADLs
- Includes mental competence considerations (these policies allow coverage when the recipient cannot perform a task due to confusion or dementia)
- Offers flexibility and choice regarding where and by whom services may be provided
- Covers a broad range of services, including skilled nursing care, intermediate care, custodial care, adult day care, home care, and respite care
- Has few (or no) exclusions for pre-existing conditions
- Does not require a hospital stay to trigger benefits
- Offers inflation protection, is guaranteed renewable, and has

"step-up" and "step-down" options (these allow the holder to change coverage as his or her needs change)

As you can see, careful shopping is key when buying a long-term-care policy. Premiums are expensive (usually $500 per month or more), and rise over time. Coverage stops when you can no longer pay premiums. (For this reason, experts recommend that premiums not exceed 5 percent of your after-tax income.) Exclusions and long waiting periods can render a policy useless for relatively brief care needs. Read the policy carefully before you buy, and get advice from a financial advisor, who can assess your holdings and determine whether you might do better investing the money you would have spent on premiums, earmarking the earnings for medical needs.

Veteran's benefits

Any United States veteran is eligible for medical care at a Veterans Affairs (VA) medical facility, whether or not their current problems are service-related. However, because there are many more veterans than beds at this time, priority is given to urgent, acute conditions. Service-related injuries and illnesses are taken next, and veterans with nonurgent problems who can afford to pay for care elsewhere are the lowest priority.

The VA runs some long-term-care facilities, but waiting lists tend to be long. Some VA centers offer in-home nursing care from their own agencies, but limitations and restrictions apply. If your loved one is eligible for veteran's benefits, it's a good idea to contact the local VA office to find out exactly what's available in the area and what services your loved one is eligible for. Be sure to ask about the VA's Special Pension Aide and Attendance program, a relatively new benefit designed to help defray the costs of in-home, assisted living, and nursing home care for veterans and their spouses (even if care needs are not service-related). Aide and Attendance benefits in 2008 topped out at $1,519 per month for a veteran, $976 per month for a surviving spouse, and $1,801 per month for a couple where both partners required services.

You can obtain information regarding veteran's benefits from the Veterans Affairs website (www.va.gov) or by calling 800-827-1000. Contact information for local veterans' services (including local VA contact information) is usually listed in the *Human Services* section of the phone book. (Look under "Veterans.")

What If We Run Out of Money?

Although there are options for funding long-term care even if you have little income and few assets, care choices narrow as funds diminish. Federal law ensures that residents cannot be discharged from facilities just because they've transferred to Medicaid coverage. However, one can be denied admission if the facility doesn't accept Medicaid or if all available Medicaid beds are filled. Finding a vacancy can be challenging, and your loved one may wind up in a facility with few amenities and a less-than-desirable location.

The bottom line: You won't be denied care if you genuinely need it, but you might have to wait a while to get it, and it won't be exactly what you wanted. Medicaid will always press for the lowest possible level of care, so your loved one will likely receive fewer services than he would if he were funding his care in other ways. It is illegal for facilities or providers to discriminate against people on the basis of funding, but the harsh reality is, you get what you pay for, and facilities funded primarily by Medicaid don't have many frills and niceties.

Must the Nursing Home Get It All?

Not necessarily. With proper advance planning, you can transfer certain assets and still be eligible for Medicaid and other benefits. However, this must be done legally and well in advance of the time you apply for Medicaid coverage. We discuss strategies for protecting one's assets in Chapter 6. You may be tempted to "hide" assets, or transfer them outside federal guidelines, but resist this temptation. If asset transfers and other financial arrangements are improper or illegal, your assets can—and will—be seized and used to pay for unreimbursed care costs after your death. Unless you follow the letter of the law, then yes—the nursing home will indeed "get it all."

6

Leaving Home for the Nursing Home: Preparing for the Dreaded Day

Lackawanna, New York; October 19, 2007. A four-hour standoff ended peacefully at 3 P.M. today, when Mr. Melvin Rittenhouse surrendered to police and mental health authorities. Mr. Rittenhouse had barricaded himself in his home at 627 Carrotwood Drive around eleven o'clock this morning, when a team of Geriatric Assessment Workers from Erie County Psychiatric Center arrived to evaluate his mental status. After being verbally threatened by Mr. Rittenhouse, Center personnel notified law enforcement officials, who arrived on the scene around 11:30 A.M.

At various times throughout the day, Mr. Rittenhouse was observed brandishing a shotgun, handgun, baseball bat, and hunting knife. Although no shots were fired, Mr. Rittenhouse leveled his shotgun on several occasions when confronted by authorities, causing police to clear the area and evacuate nearby homes. Mr. Rittenhouse finally surrendered his weapons and exited his trailer home after a lengthy telephone discussion with his daughter, Shirley Rittenhouse Melby, also of Lackawanna. The content of that discussion remains unknown at this time.

Described by nearby residents as a "loner," but a "good, quiet neighbor," Melvin Rittenhouse had recently started to exhibit behaviors described by his daughter as "alarming" and "dangerous." She reports that on two occasions during the past month, Mr. Rittenhouse was seen walking down the center of Route 414; on both occasions, he was detained by officers of the State Police, and returned to his home. On a third occasion, one week ago, Mr. Rittenhouse attempted to enter a local convenience store wearing only his bathrobe and bedroom slippers.

Mr. Rittenhouse's daughter reports that she had encouraged him to seek treatment for his current difficulties numerous times during the past several weeks, but that he repeatedly refused all offers of help.

Center officials declined to discuss the outcome of Mr. Rittenhouse's evaluation and would neither confirm nor deny that he is currently a patient at the facility. However, Sergeant William Tucker of the New York State Police issued a brief statement early this evening indicating that Mr. Rittenhouse is "no longer a threat" to local residents. Mr. Rittenhouse's brother and sister-in-law have taken up temporary residence in his trailer home, safeguarding his possessions and trying to restore order to the residence, which sister-in-law Amanda Delfreesio described as "cluttered," "dirty," and "filled with trash."

Believe it or not, an incident like this actually happened a few years ago. There's little chance that you'll encounter something so dramatic as this (Mr. Rittenhouse obviously had psychological problems to begin with), but one thing is for sure: You *will* encounter roadblocks—either now or later—if you do not prepare adequately for your loved one's impending move to a nursing home.

What must be done? Several things. You must decide what to bring to the nursing home and what to leave behind. You must make sure your loved one's legal and financial affairs are in order. You must prepare the house to avoid damage, deterioration, and theft. And last—but certainly not least—you must help your loved one prepare for the move, psychologically and emotionally. That's where we'll begin.

Psychological Preparations

Several years ago, researchers studying stressful life events asked people to assign point values to different experiences, with higher point values reflecting greater subjective stress and disruption. Moving ("changing residences") received one of the highest of all stress scores—higher even than trouble at work and certain violations of the law.

If moving to a new home is stressful under ordinary circumstances, imagine how disruptive moving to a nursing home can be. No surprise, then, that as the "dreaded day" draws near, your loved one's difficulties may become even more pronounced—stress will do that. His cognitive functions may deteriorate, and his problematic behaviors may worsen. He might become much more emotional, or perhaps close up and show no emotion at all.

These are all normal, predictable reactions to an impending nursing home move, but they may still cause problems when moving day arrives. You can minimize difficulties by doing two things. First, talk with your loved one about his fears and concerns—let him unburden himself and tell you what's worrying him. Second, know what sorts of last-minute surprises you might encounter on moving day, so you can plan for them.

Discussing last-minute fears and concerns

Even if you and your loved one have discussed the plan at length, you should still expect some last-minute concerns to emerge. Here are three common ones, and some useful responses:

- *What if I hate it there?* If your loved one raises this issue, be honest: Acknowledge that at first, he might. It will be strange and unfamiliar, perhaps even a bit frightening. Your loved one's first thought when he arrives may be that this was a big mistake, and he wants out—now! Warn him ahead of time that he might feel this way and remind him that like anything new, the only way to find out if this arrangement will work is to give it a chance. Agree on a reasonable period (a month or two is good), and tell your loved one that if it really doesn't seem to be working at that point, you'll reconvene and come up with a new plan.
- *I won't know anybody....* This might be true, particularly if the move is rapid (like a transfer from a hospital). If your loved one has had the chance to meet some of the staff or residents in advance, remind him of welcoming statements from the visit ("Remember, Dad, how Mrs. Smith said she was hoping you'd join her bridge group?"). You can also remind your loved one of the things he can offer others—skills and talents that will make

him a valued member of the community ("Dad, you know how people open up to you—you'll know everything about everyone in the building!").

• *What if it's too...?* Everyone's got a few pet peeves—noise, the wrong food, bad TV. No matter how many times you reassure your loved one, those concerns will linger until he gets to experience things for himself. Still, you might be able to do a little table-turning to defuse the situation temporarily: Use the same reassurances your loved one used on you when you were afraid of something new ("Remember what you told me when I was afraid to go to summer camp/a new job/my first apartment?").

Avoiding last-minute surprises

These are frustrating, but less so if you anticipate them and prepare ahead of time. Three last-minute glitches are particularly problematic. Though rare, you should be aware of:

• *The breakdown.* When you spoke on the phone this morning, Mom seemed OK. Now she's a wreck—screaming, crying... just falling apart. She's steadfastly refusing to leave the house, and when you press the issue, she gets even more agitated. The key question here is, have you seen this before? Is this your loved one's habitual response to not getting her way? If she is genuinely agitated, your best strategy is to soothe her and try to calm her down. However, if this is just her way of intimidating you, you should proceed in a businesslike manner and not reinforce her manipulative behavior.

• *The slowdown.* All of a sudden, your loved one's vocabulary has dwindled to three responses: "Yes," "No," and "I don't know." It took her five minutes to put on her coat, and now that it's on, she needs to go to the bathroom. You're already late—and getting later by the minute. What to do? First of all, stay calm. Call the facility, advise them that you're behind schedule and continue your attempts to proceed at a normal pace. Make it clear to your loved one that stalling won't change the plan—you're going to get there, even if it takes all day.

• *The sabotage.* You show up at Mom's house, only to find Cousin

Bert loading her bags into his car—he's found another, "better" nursing home, and he's bringing her there, whether you like it or not. This is where your united front of family members comes in handy. Let Cousin Bert know that the group's decision stands— he has no right to interfere. If necessary, bring in other family members to reinforce the message. Gang up on him if you have to—few of us have the wherewithal to oppose a group of people who tell us in no uncertain terms that we're out of line.

What to Pack (and Leave Behind)

What you'll bring to the home-away-from-home is dictated by the setting and the person's care needs. Keep in mind that as care plans change, brief moves may turn into longer ones (or vice versa), and you'll have to adjust accordingly.

The rule of thumb here is simple: Your loved one should bring enough to satisfy her immediate needs, but not much more than that. Space is at a premium in most assisted living, group home, and nursing home settings, and extra storage space is hard to come by. You'll probably have to fit everything into one closet and a couple of bureaus, so start out relatively sparse, storing off-season clothing and other non-essentials elsewhere. You can bring them to the facility later, as needed.

Space limitations aside, certain items are essential for every nursing home resident. Many nursing homes will provide a list of suggested items, so ask ahead of time. You can also use the What to Bring to the Nursing Home checklist starting on page 243 to ensure you don't forget anything important. Key items include:

Clothing

This can be remarkably tricky. If your loved one has spent a lifetime in a house without air conditioning, she might find the August chill of the average long-term-care facility unsettling. (Bring extra sweaters.) If housedresses are her preferred garb, but she's scheduled to spend time doing leg stretches in physical therapy, sweatpants and sneakers are in order. Ask facility staff what clothes she'll need—they have experience and can give good advice. Go through your loved one's wardrobe in advance, and fill in any missing pieces. For some folks, a preparatory shopping trip can be a fun transitional activity.

HOW NOT TO DEAL WITH THE NURSING HOME ISSUE

Once up
skirted t
loved o
leave—p
posed to
they've t
jungle o
ing" mig
loved or
ample, i
facility),

to upset Mom"
would invite their
rsing home and
always been op-
-dumping"), and
ugh a paperwork
, "granny-dump-
. Deceiving your
s wrong (for ex-
admitted to the

Clothing
son needs ext
needs more r
culty handling
are needed he
for a trip to a
celebratory di

. An incontinent per-
rts. A bedfast person
rokes may have diffi-
d clothing protectors
tfit that's appropriate
e to wear to a special
ively brief stay).

All nursi
enjoy ha
they are

home residents
are popular, as
ited dexterity. If
you do consider bringing a television along, be realistic—a four-foot-wide flat-screen TV won't fit in most rooms. And if you do opt for private television, you'll need to have cable service set up for the resident ahead of time. The nursing home can help with this, though you pay for the service itself.

The same goes for the telephone: All nursing homes have public phones, but many residents like having their own phone as well. (Again, this is an additional out-of-pocket cost.) If you go this route, consider purchasing an easy-to-dial model with large, lighted buttons, and don't forget to have phone service activated in the resident's room. Although cell phones might seem like a good option, many facilities ban them due to the possibility of loss, theft, interference with medical equipment, and privacy violations (most cell phones have cameras).

The right shoes are important. Many facilities prohibit walking barefoot, so slippers are essential. If your loved one will be in rehab for a broken hip or learning to walk again after a stroke, he'll need nonslip walking shoes or sneakers. The physical therapist will have an opinion about proper footwear and should be consulted ahead of time.

Most facilities provide laundry services for residents, and they get pretty adept at knowing what belongs to whom, thanks to labeling systems and laundry bags. Be realistic, however, and expect that some items will be lost and some ruined in the wash. It's a good idea to choose easy-care clothing. Delicate items requiring special treatment don't hold up well to institutional laundering.

THE DRESS WITH LEGS

The resident was talking about her granddaughter's upcoming wedding, and when I asked what she planned to wear, she frowned.

"I don't know," she said. "My dress walked away."

"Your dress walked away?"

"Yes, my daughter bought me a beautiful two-piece outfit for Christmas. I had it right there in the closet, but when April called to tell me about the wedding, I looked for the bag and it was gone."

"Could it have gotten lost in the laundry?" I asked.

"No, I was saving it. I hadn't worn it yet."

At some point every day, all nursing home residents vacate their rooms so maintenance and housekeeping staff can do repairs and cleaning. Most rooms have a single locking drawer, and locks tend to be generic and easily opened, since forgetful residents frequently misplace their keys. Occasionally a confused resident will wander into someone else's room, mistaking it for her own, and take what she assumes to be her stuff. Worse, not everyone who walks the halls is honest, and in any given day a veritable army of consultants, technicians, delivery people, sales reps, and visitors files through. It's impossible for nursing home security to keep a close eye on everyone.

Bringing up the issue of theft with staff is almost certain to elicit a defensive reaction, so if something goes missing try to be firm but polite. Don't accuse, but do keep asking questions until you get some reasonable answers. And to prevent problems from occurring down the line, ask about labeling procedures, secure locks for drawers and closets, and facility policies regarding the replacement of "missing laundry" and other items.

Toiletries

Many facilities provide basic toiletries for short stays, but most expect the resident to bring her own shampoo, bath products, makeup, and incontinence products. An important exception concerns products used to maintain skin integrity in people confined to beds or wheelchairs. For medical reasons, the doctor might want to specify which of these products the patient uses.

A good rule of thumb is to begin with average amounts of those toiletries the person usually uses during a two-week period, and add or remove items as the person's needs become clear. Don't buy giant economy sizes until you know whether there's sufficient storage space. In most nursing homes, there won't be.

Familiar items

Again, space limitations may dictate what is feasible. Most nursing home living spaces will accommodate favorite pictures, a telephone, a television, a few dozen books, and a radio or "talking book" player. Some will accommodate a well-loved chair and one or two other small pieces of furniture. Use special caution where irreplaceable, fragile, and valuable items are concerned. Things get broken in care facilities, and sadly, things get stolen as well.

If the resident simply can't live without something fragile or valuable, do what you can to ensure the item's safety. Pictures can be secured to walls. Knickknacks can be displayed in locked, sturdy cases bolted to a shelf or desktop. Remember, though, that no matter how many precautions you take, some things may be damaged or lost. If the resident has been planning to pass along a valued object to someone, this might be a good time to do so. She can always "visit" the cherished object during off-grounds trips, and she might rest easier knowing that it's safe.

Orienting cues

Most facilities are sensitive to the disorienting effect of being in a new setting, and they provide numerous cues to remind the resident where she is, what time it is, what she's doing next, etc. Clocks, calendars, and schedules (both daily and monthly) are often permanent fixtures in residents' rooms. If the facility doesn't provide these things, buy them on your own and personalize them for the resident. (For example, mark calendars with family members' birthdays, anniversaries, etc.)

WHAT ABOUT FOOD IN THE RESIDENT'S ROOM?

Having some favorite snacks nearby can be comforting to the resident. It's one more familiar thing in an unfamiliar place and can go a long way toward helping the person feel at home.

If you intend to bring some snacks along on move-in day, be sure to check with the facility first. Most nursing homes allow residents to keep treats in their rooms (as long as there's no medical reason not to), but most facilities have rules about appropriate food storage. If asked, many facilities will be glad to provide refrigeration or safe food storage in an accessible area near the resident's room.

Legal Preparations

Several legal documents should be in place before your loved one enters any long-term-care facility. Many nursing homes actually require that some of these documents be prepared prior to admission. If you haven't completed these documents beforehand, admissions staff may ask you to sign "boilerplate" versions of them when you arrive at the facility. Key legal documents for the nursing home resident include:

Last will and testament

Sometimes referred to simply as a *will*, this is a document that formalizes a person's wishes concerning the disposition of property, guardianship of minor children, and administration of the estate after his or her death. A will can help preserve assets for one's heirs by minimizing fees and taxes. However, a will does not enable one to avoid *probate* (the court-supervised proceedings that formally conclude a person's legal and financial matters after death). In fact, a will is essentially a written set of instructions for the probate court (hence, it can speed the probate process considerably). A nursing home will not keep a copy of the resident's will on file, but they will want a list of people who should be contacted in case of death, and that list usually includes the *executor*—the person responsible for handling the will and managing the probate process.

Advance directives

Advance directives are documents that formalize a person's wishes regarding future medical care and name an individual (or individuals) to make treatment decisions on his or her behalf. These are essential to the nursing home. The resident may refuse to stipulate his choices in both of these areas, but if he does, he will be advised of the potential costs and consequences. If the resident chooses not to complete these documents, this fact is noted in the file, and state law regarding decision-making prevails.

Most advance directives take one of two forms: the *health care proxy* and *the living will*.

- *A Health Care Proxy* (also called a *Durable Power of Attorney for Health Care*) delegates decision-making ability about medical matters to another individual, called a *proxy*. The language used in a health care proxy should be as specific as possible—some states have disallowed health care proxies that were overly vague or ambiguous. In addition, the document should be in place before your loved one undergoes any significant medical procedure. Older adults often emerge from surgery in a state of *delirium* (chemically induced confusion and agitation), and they need someone to make health care decisions for them until they regain their bearings. The health care proxy should be on file in the nursing home, the office of the patient's primary physician, and any facility where the person is undergoing a medical procedure. (The nursing home is responsible for sending this information along with the resident if he or she needs out-of-facility care, but you should still advise other care providers

THE NATIONAL ACADEMY OF ELDER LAW ATTORNEYS

If you can use local contacts to find a good, reputable attorney experienced in elder law, by all means do so. If you need help in locating an attorney to assist with your legal and financial preparations, or simply want to obtain useful, up-to-date information on elder law, contact the National Academy of Elder Law Attorneys by mail (1604 North Country Club Road, Tucson, AZ, 85716), telephone (520-881-4005), or via the Internet (www.naela.org).

yourself, to decrease the likelihood of errors.)

- *A Living Will* (also called a *Directive to Physicians*) outlines a person's choices regarding extraordinary measures taken to prolong life when death is imminent. The person may choose which procedures they will and will not accept. Although the person cannot ask that active measures be taken to end her life, she may decide whether she wants to be on life support equipment such as ventilators or feeding tubes. The "imminence" of death is key here—the living will goes into effect *only* when physicians rule that the person is likely to die in the very near future. For a living will to be effective, it must be written in very specific language; vague or ambiguous wording can raise so many questions that the document becomes invalid. The care receiver's primary physician and health care proxy should both have copies, and a copy should also be on file in the nursing home itself. And remember: Laws surrounding living wills vary from state to state, so check with your attorney early in the process.

Power of attorney

This is a legal document through which one person (the *principal*) authorizes another person (the *agent* or *attorney-in-fact*) to act on his or her behalf. To stay in effect when the principal becomes unable to manage his or her own affairs, the document must be a *durable power of attorney*. (A regular power of attorney is automatically invalidated when the principal becomes incapacitated.) Nursing homes don't insist that the resident appoint a durable power of attorney, but they strongly recommend it, because it makes life easier for everyone if the resident becomes unable to manage his or her financial affairs. The nursing home will keep a copy of the document on file, so they know who to contact when decisions must be made.

A durable power of attorney can be as broad or narrow as one chooses. It can allow the agent to perform all financial tasks for the principal or simply enable the agent to pay bills, sign checks, or carry out other specific tasks named in the document. Your loved one must decide ahead of time how broad or narrow she wants the power of attorney to be: Once the principal becomes incapacitated, a durable power of attorney is exceedingly difficult to change, except through a lengthy and expensive court proceeding.

Keep in mind that a durable power of attorney does not forbid the principal

THE TRAGEDY OF TERRI SCHIAVO

If only she had put advance directives in place, none of us would ever have heard of Terri Schiavo, and the battle between her parents and ex-husband would not have played itself out night after night on the news. Every tragedy brings with it a lesson, and this one did too.

Unknown wishes are impossible to honor, and in an emergency situation workers don't stop to ask about DNR papers. A number of states are working to ensure that an individual's wishes regarding treatment will be respected by establishing uniform communication tools that specify that person's decisions. For example, New York State is implementing the Medical Orders for Life-Sustaining Treatment (MOLST) form project, in which a hard-to-miss hot pink form must accompany the person during any hospitalization, transfer, or procedure performed at an outside provider's office. The form specifies the patient's preferences regarding such matters as CPR, ventilation, intubation, artificial hydration and nutrition, use of antibiotics, and hospital transfers.

People's preferences change over time, of course, so the MOLST must be reviewed in a discussion between the patient (or her proxy) and physician whenever certain health changes occur, or at specified intervals. The physician is required to document the outcome of these discussions in writing, and to update the MOLST form accordingly. While a properly used MOLST form will be a much-edited document, it can go a long way toward ensuring proper care, and peace of mind.

from performing the tasks named in the document—it simply identifies another person who may *also* perform them. A durable power of attorney should be executed as soon as possible, because if your loved one becomes incapacitated without this document in place, a rather complex court procedure will be needed to accomplish the same thing. (One important caveat: If your loved one has assets in two or more states, she will need a separate power of attorney for each state.)

Funeral Arrangements

Most nursing homes require that you provide basic information regarding funeral arrangements prior to admission. The timing couldn't be worse, of course. (Think of the message this sends to the resident!) Nonetheless, the requirement is there, and here's what you'll be asked when your loved one is admitted to the facility:

- *The name of the resident's mortician*—the person who'll be managing their funeral arrangements. You may be asked to produce written proof (a letter from the mortician) that this arrangement has been made. The resident is permitted to change to a different mortician after admission.
- *Whether the resident has a prepaid burial or cremation plan*—an arrangement regarding where the service will be held, what type of casket or urn will be used, what clothes the person will be buried or cremated in, and so forth.
- *Whether the resident has a prepaid burial plot,* and if so, where it's located.
- *Any special funeral instructions.* If your loved one has special needs related to religious beliefs or personal preferences, these should be specified.

Financial Preparations

Living expenses continue after a person enters a nursing home—especially if the person chooses to hold on to her house and/or car while she's away. It is important to make certain financial preparations prior to entering a nursing home.

Budgets

Even if your loved one never worked out a formal budget for managing her living costs, you should. You can use the Monthly Income and Expenses Worksheet starting on page 247 to do this. If expenses exceed income, the person will have to: (a) find new income sources, (b) trim expenses, or (c) do both. (Sometimes a combined strategy works best.) If you uncover a serious budget shortfall here, it may be time for another family meeting.

Banking, bills, and taxes

Here's where a durable power of attorney comes in handy. If the person still owns a house or car, the agent can make the necessary payments without involving the nursing home resident. Income tax forms and Social Security paperwork can be completed by the agent, if need be. The agent can also deal with nursing home bills. If the resident still owns her home, be sure that bills go there or to the home of the power of attorney. (It's not a good idea to forward bills to the nursing home.) If payments can be made electronically, through automatic withdrawals from a checking account, you might want to explore this option.

The importance of keeping good records can't be overstated. For one thing, the principal and the courts have the right to review the agent's work at any time. And some nursing home residents find it comforting to review the agent's records, just to see that everything is in order. Unless your loved one is adamant about not wanting to be bothered, or her mental state suggests against it, it's a good idea to schedule periodic review sessions where you go over this information together. Keep the information well-organized and accessible, and don't rely on memory to determine whether something was paid. If someone else ever has to take over, he or she won't know what's been done if it wasn't recorded properly.

Continue to deposit income checks (investments, pension, Social Security, Medicaid, etc.) into the resident's bank account or arrange for these to be deposited directly. Keep bank accounts active by making a small deposit into each account at least once every six months. (A dollar or two will do.) Dormant bank accounts become the property of the state after a certain amount of time has passed (though the amount of time differs from state to state.)

KATRINA'S LEGACY

One of the most disturbing images from Hurricane Katrina in 2005 was the rows of wheelchair-bound nursing home residents stranded in stifling facilities, with no way for authorities to move them to safer quarters. After this catastrophe, many nursing homes developed detailed emergency evacuation plans, or refined and updated existing ones. Administrators in a number of high-risk areas periodically hold formal "disaster drills" to hone the effectiveness of their plans.

If your loved one is in a high-risk area for hurricanes or other natural disasters, you may be asked about your family's plans for evacuation in the event of emergency, and whether you wish to delegate evacuation responsibility to the facility or plan to do it yourself. Think carefully about the pros and cons of both options, and talk with nursing home officials before making a final decision.

CERTIFIED FINANCIAL PLANNERS

You should always use a Certified Financial Planner to help with asset management (yours and your loved one's). To use this title, the person must have undergone appropriate professional training and must also attend periodic continuing education seminars to stay up-to-date with changes in tax laws and other relevant matters.

You can find Certified Financial Planners in the Yellow Pages of your phone book. (Look under "Financial Planning Consultants.") Two national associations can also help steer you toward reputable professionals and provide information regarding the financial planning process. These are:

The Financial Planning Association*
800-322-4237
www.fpanet.org

The Society of Financial Service Professionals
17 Campus Boulevard, Suite 201
Newtown Square, PA 19073
610-526-2500
www.financialpro.org

*Because the Financial Planning Association has headquarters in different areas of the country, there is no central mailing address for inquiries. (Telephone and Internet contact is best.)

Asset management

Asset management is a lifelong task, and if this is the first time your loved one has dealt with the issue, the situation will not be ideal—certain asset management options might no longer be available, given your loved one's circumstances. Even if your loved one has been an obsessive money-manager for many years, it's a good idea to consult with a certified financial planner at this point and an attorney experienced in elder law.

The first step in asset management involves calculating the person's *net worth*—the total amount of her assets, minus liabilities (what is owed). We've provided a worksheet for this on page 250, and even if your loved one has calculated her net worth already, you should probably do it again. You can catch mistakes by doing this (and besides, things have changed now that your loved one is entering a nursing home).

Your financial planner can give you advice regarding asset management—strategies for preserving your loved one's assets so as many as possible can be passed on to others. One important issue, of course, involves preserving your loved one's assets in the face of substantial medical and nursing home bills. (We discussed this issue in Chapter 5.) It is also important to be aware of the impact of estate taxes on assets passed on to others. The first $3.5 million of anyone's estate is currently excluded from estate taxes through the *estate tax exemption,* but the estate tax is expected to be repealed in 2010. Three and a half million dollars sounds like a lot of money, but many people are surprised when they discover how many assets their loved ones actually have (and how much they lose to Uncle Sam when inheritance time comes—currently 45 cents of every dollar over the exempted amount).

A will is one of the most widely used asset management tools, but by itself, a will is an ineffective way of protecting one's estate. Here are three other strategies you should know about:

- *Gifts.* According to 2007 IRS guidelines, a person may give an unlimited number of recipients cash gifts of up to $12,000 per year, and the recipients of those gifts don't owe a penny in tax. Even if the same person receives $12,000 each year for ten—or even fifty—years, that person still owes no tax whatsoever on the gifts—they are not counted as income. Two spouses can give $12,000 each to the same person, so it's possible for a couple to give a total of $48,000 each year to their child and his spouse ($12,000 each to the child and $12,000 each to the spouse) without triggering any sort of tax event.
- *Trusts.* A trust is a legal entity used to hold money, property, and other assets. Trusts come in many forms, and most are quite complicated. At this point, you'll likely be dealing with a "living trust." ("Testamentary trusts" are established after a person dies.) But even here, you must choose between a *revocable living trust* and an *irrevocable living trust.* The best advice we can give you is to consult with experts before you make a move in this arena. It is virtually impossible to set up a trust properly without the advice of an attorney and financial planner. True, you'll have to pay some fairly hefty consulting fees, but it's worth it—you'll save money in the long run.

• *Joint ownership.* Married couples typically own their house and other assets (such as bank accounts and investments) as *joint tenants with rights of survivorship.* The advantage of this from a financial standpoint is that all property owned in this manner passes immediately to the surviving spouse when one spouse dies—these assets are not subjected to probate, and they are immune from estate tax. Two people need not be married to establish joint ownership—parents sometimes own a house jointly with one or more of their children—but be warned: Laws surrounding joint ownership between unmarried people vary from state to state. (Check with a financial planner on this.) Be sure not to confuse *joint ownership with rights of survivorship* with *ownership as tenants in common.* In the latter situation, there are no rights of survivorship and very different tax consequences. Both setups have certain advantages, and a financial planner can help you decide which one is right for you.

SHARE THE WEALTH—AND RESPONSIBILITY FOR MANAGING IT

The research findings are clear: When one member of a couple becomes seriously ill, those couples who shared responsibility for managing finances throughout their marriage fare better than those wherein one person (usually the husband) handled all the money matters. Unfortunately, only 11 percent of couples use this share-the-responsibility approach to investing and bill paying, so it is not unusual for the healthier partner—usually the woman—to be at a loss regarding financial issues when the lifelong money manager becomes ill.

If your loved one finds herself in this situation, the first thing to do is gather as much financial information as possible. If an accountant prepared the couple's taxes, this will help; if a financial planner managed their investments, even better—the records will be more up-to-date and more detailed. Help your loved one work through the different elements of the couple's shared finances: bills to be paid, investments to be monitored, bank accounts and CDs, outstanding loans and mortgages. If the financial picture is simple, you and your loved one may be able to work through it together. If it's complex, it might be worth contacting a Certified Financial Planner to help organize the situation and recommend how best to proceed.

Preparing the House

Whether occupied or empty, houses need care. The grass grows, the leaves fall, time and weather take their toll. When a house is unoccupied, rodents and other critters (sometimes of the human variety) find their way in, and rearrange things to fit their own needs. You'll definitely need to prepare the house for your loved one's nursing home stay, but the *way* you prepare it will depend upon whether or not someone will remain in the home during the care receiver's absence.

If the house will be unoccupied

If a short-term nursing home stay is anticipated, prepare the house as if you were going on an extended vacation. Put newspaper delivery and trash pickup services on hold. Arrange to have mail forwarded or held at the post office. Have voice mail forwarded, or check it periodically. Advise "automatic delivery" fuel oil providers that the house will be shut down for a while; they'll reduce deliveries accordingly. Provide a phone number that providers can call if there's an emergency.

Stopping services altogether might sound attractive, but think before you act: The costs of re-establishing services can sometimes be prohibitive, especially if a stay proves shorter than expected. Only terminate services if the amount of money you save exceeds the start-up costs you'll pay later on. And keep in mind that some things can't be re-established the exact same way once they're discontinued. For example, if you stop phone service there's no guarantee you'll get the old number back when you start the service up again (an important consideration for someone who has had the same phone number for many years).

Shutting down a house completely is rarely a good idea. Water or drainage pipes can freeze in winter, resulting in costly repairs. A house without air conditioning or dehumidification may develop mold and insect problems in warm weather. Your best bet is to keep heat and air conditioning going at minimal levels—but do keep them going. If you're unsure how to proceed, ask service representatives from various utilities for advice, or consult a local realtor.

If the house doesn't have an alarm system, this might be the time to have one installed. Because it's considered a home improvement, an alarm system is an acceptable expense under current Medicaid disbursement rules. If you can't afford an alarm, ask a trusted neighbor to check the place regularly—or do it yourself, if you live nearby. Arrange to have the grass cut and the sidewalk shoveled so the house looks occupied, and put some lights, plus a TV or radio, on a variable-schedule timer.

Go through the cupboards, and get rid of perishable foods. Check garages and basement storage areas for flammable materials, and store them appropriately, or discard them. Drain the gas tanks of snowblowers, lawnmowers, and other equipment that will remain idle for an extended period. If a car must be stored, check with your mechanic regarding how best to do this.

If someone will remain in the home

This makes your task easier, but certain things still must be done. If the remaining occupant has lived in the home but never helped maintain it, she will have to learn fast. Most important, the occupant must learn basic emergency procedures—what to do if the power goes out, how to turn off the water main in the event of a leak, where to find the electrical circuit box. Go through the house with her, taking notes and making "what to do" lists that can be accessed easily in an emergency. A "who to call" list with names and phone numbers should also be available to the occupant. Keep one copy of this list in the house, give another to a trusted neighbor, and make sure your loved one's power of attorney has a copy as well.

Some tasks look easy until you try to do them, so insist that the person try now, not later. Together, the two of you can make a "practice run," checking unfamiliar equipment to see what will need to be tuned up or replaced, and what tasks might have to be delegated to others. If the occupant can't operate the old push mower but can run a riding mower with ease, consider buying one. If the occupant can't push the snowblower around the driveway, arrange to have a plowing service clear the path.

In addition to the physical challenges, there are some psychological aspects of living alone that people don't always anticipate. Handling things alone is tougher than many people realize—especially if they haven't lived alone before. The lone occupant must now structure his or her own day, and schedule things (like meals) that were once scheduled for them. The very idea of "aloneness" can be frightening, and oftentimes people develop a "why bother?" attitude with respect to things like shopping or cooking (or bathing or shaving). When someone you love needs nursing home care, it's easy to forget about the spouse or sibling they left behind, but don't. This person needs your support as well, but given the current situation, he or she might not be comfortable asking for it. Don't wait to be asked: Offer instead.

7

Anxicty, Anger, Fear, and Guilt: Adjusting to the New Situation

"John? Is that you?"

"What? I'm not...who is this?"

"It's me, John. It's Dad."

"Dad? What's going on? Is something wrong?"

"No, no. Nothing like that."

"Dad, for cryin' out loud, do you know what time it is? It's two o'clock in the morning!"

"I know. I'm sorry. It's just that...I needed to talk to you."

"Now?"

"John, I'm scared."

"How's that, Dad? Scared of what?"

"I don't know. Nothing. Everything."

"What do you mean, Dad?"

"I don't know. It's just...nothing feels right. I can't sleep. It feels strange to be here. It doesn't feel like home."

"It hasn't gotten any better? Since last week, I mean?"

"To tell you the truth, no. It's even a little worse, maybe, since yesterday. I didn't tell you—I got a roommate.

"The two of you don't get along?"

"No, no—nothing like that. It's just strange is all. Having another person in the room, I mean."

"Oh."

"It's not his fault. He's very nice. It's just that I wake up at night and hear him breathing, and…I think for a minute…it's almost like your mother's back. But then I realize where I am, and what's going on, and I get scared."

"Maybe you'll start to get used to it, Dad. Isn't that what the nurse told us on Friday? She said this kind of thing happens. They expect it. It's normal."

"I know that, John, but it's not normal for *me*."

"I'm sorry."

"No, it's not your fault. It's just…what should I do?"

"Well, is that nurse on tonight?"

"Ms. Freeman? I think so. Why?"

"Why don't you go talk to her?"

"No, I couldn't. I don't want to bother her."

"Dad, what did she say when you spoke to her last week?"

"I know, John, but still…"

"C'mon, Dad. She said to come see her if you had trouble sleeping. She said that, right? I was there."

"Yeah, but…"

"She wouldn't have said it if she didn't mean it, right?"

"I suppose."

"Go talk to her, Dad. Sit by the TV for a while. Don't just fret—you'll feel better if you do something."

"OK. All right."

"Seriously, Dad. I mean it. You promise?"

"Yes. Yes, I promise. I can see her there behind the desk. I'll go over as soon as we hang up."

"Seriously, Dad…"

"All right, all right. You know, John, you can be a real nudge when you want to be."

"Hey, well…some things never change."

"Good-bye, son. Thanks."

"Bye, Dad. I'll see you tomorrow after work, OK?"

"OK, John. I'll see you then."

You've devoted an enormous amount of time and effort to finding the best possible situation for your loved one. You put your own needs on hold, took on new and unfamiliar challenges, and dealt with some very unpleasant realities. Now your loved one has taken up residence in a nursing home, and you're looking forward to some closure, a well-deserved rest, and a pat on the back for all your hard work.

Hold on just a minute, and take a deep breath. Closure's not coming—at least not just yet. There's work left to be done to ensure that your loved one's transition to the nursing home goes as smoothly as possible. In this chapter, we discuss the nursing home adjustment process from both caregiver and care receiver perspectives. We go over the nuts-and-bolts of visits and off-grounds trips, as well as strategies for maintaining telephone, mail, and e-mail contact with your loved one.

Common Reactions to Placing a Family Member in a Nursing Home

Caregivers experience a range of emotions when a parent, spouse, or sibling moves to a nursing home. Some of these reactions are predictable; others are surprising. Expect to experience some—maybe all—of the following:

- *Fear and anxiety.* In Chapter 6, we discussed how frightening nursing home placement can be to the care receiver. You'll probably experience some anxiety as well, expecially during those first few days, until you're confident that staff can handle the situation. As time passes, and you discover that the nursing home can deal with minor glitches and more serious setbacks, your fear and anxiety will subside.
- *Sadness and depression.* Placing a family member in a nursing home involves loss. Even if your loved one lives for many more

years, a phase of his life has ended and a new one has begun. He is not the person he used to be, and neither are you. You may find yourself experiencing periods of sadness, tearfulness—even mild depression. This is normal. It is part of the mourning process. Don't deny it or hurry it out the door. That will just prolong the agony.

- *Guilt and shame.* When sadness arrives, guilt and shame usually follow. You might experience guilt at having "abandoned" your loved one or shame at what a "bad person" you are for not being a more devoted caregiver. Trying to talk yourself out of these feelings won't work (feelings aren't rational enough to be argued with like that). Instead, consider joining a support group for family members of nursing home patients. (We discussed strategies for locating these groups in Chapter 1.)

- *Anger and resentment.* Now that nursing home placement is complete, you'll encounter renewed pressure on other fronts. The children who tolerated your absence while you searched for a home care worker suddenly grow impatient and start clamoring for your attention. The spouse who listened politely while you obsessed about placement settings hints that he'd rather not hear another word about Mom's arthritis. Everyone seems to think you're loaded with free time now, and they all want a piece of it. Don't be surprised if these demands cause you to feel resentful. You might become angry at those around you, or maybe at the care receiver, who'll wonder what she's done to deserve this.

- *Relief.* Expect to feel relief at least twice during the nursing home placement process: First, right after you drop off the care receiver at the nursing home, then again later on, after sadness, guilt, and anger have faded. The first relief won't last: It's a short-term response to the end of a crisis. The second relief is more permanent—it reflects your growing confidence that you've done the right thing, and the solution seems to be working.

Adjusting to the Nursing Home: The Resident's Perspective

As difficult as this transition is for you, you can be certain it's even harder for the care receiver, whose life has been turned upside down. Every person adjusts to change in his own way, but for most new nursing home residents, this adjustment period can be divided into three phases.

The arrival

The typical nursing home has a huge cast of characters—residents, three shifts' worth of staff, visitors, outside consultants, and assorted others. The new resident will meet a lot of people in a very short time. While this is exciting, it can also be overwhelming. To make the task more manageable, try to determine who your loved one will have the most contact with during the next few days and help him connect with those people first. And reassure your loved one that it will get easier with time—nobody gets all the names straight the first time around.

Three tasks you must manage on moving day:

- *Personalizing personal space.* Although people expect that the moving-in process will take a long time, it's usually done in an hour or two. Keep in mind that you're working with a fairly small space, and the locations of some large items are predetermined. (The bed must be next to the call bell and medical equipment hookups.) Once moveable furniture is placed, all you have to do is unpack clothing and toiletries and add personal touches. Most rooms in nursing homes have hooks or shelves to accommodate artwork and photos. Many nursing homes also have bulletin boards in each room for posting the resident's schedule (they'll provide this) and other information. In some facilities, staff leave greetings or invitations on the margins of the board if they stop by while the resident is out—a pleasant surprise when the resident returns.
- *Getting off on the right foot with staff.* Nursing home staff greet new folks every day, and they're good at helping nervous people settle

in to an unfamiliar environment. Rest assured, they've seen every possible resident reaction—crying, yelling, throwing up…you name it. They're virtually shock-proof. They will, however, remember this day very clearly, so take care: You might be stressed and cranky by the end of the move, but don't take it out on the staff. As the saying goes, you never get a second chance to make a first impression. No matter how bad you feel, treat staff like colleagues, not servants. Introduce yourself to each person you meet, and listen to what they say. Feel free to ask questions, but be aware that staff might not be able to answer them fully until they know your loved one better. You'll have the chance to ask these questions again in care planning meetings down the line.

• *Saying goodbye to your loved one.* Once the move is done, don't linger. Stick around for a few minutes—an hour at most—then leave. The settling-in process can't really begin until you're gone. However you're feeling, keep your good-byes casual and brief. This is not the time for tearful "I'll miss you" speeches that agitate your loved one. If you're going to cry, take it outside. You won't be the first person to break down in the social worker's office, restroom, or parking lot. But don't do it in front of your loved one.

MOVING-DAY CABLE AND TELEPHONE GLITCHES

Because private telephone and cable TV services are coordinated by outside companies—not the facility—they tend to be the arrangements most likely to glitch on moving day, especially if your loved one arrives on a weekend. Double-check with the phone and cable companies as moving day draws near, but if you arrive to find that promised services haven't materialized, don't panic. The facility has dealt with this before, and they'll arrange for your loved one to use a house phone or watch TV in a lounge until the new services begin.

The settling-in period

Adjusting to a new home is challenging at any age—even more so if the person is older. The settling-in period can vary from a week or two to several months or more. Expect this period to be longer if your loved one hasn't moved in many years, and shorter if she's moved frequently and is used to the process. Ironically, serious illness can actually ease the initial transition—people distracted by health problems tend to be less disrupted by new surroundings.

As family members turn their attention back to other areas of their lives, the new nursing home resident may experience a bit of a letdown. No longer the center of everyone's attention, the person is expected to get on with the business of adjusting to her new world. Most do just that—they make new friends, develop new routines, and settle into their new home. But some people have trouble adjusting. A few will experience prolonged bouts of homesickness; others complain about being ignored.

If asked, the majority of older folks in new settings will give a surprisingly balanced assessment of the situation. Having a broken hip stinks, they'll say, but the physical therapist is nice. Having a roommate isn't fun, but the food's pretty good. Harried family members tend to pick up on one side of the equation or the other: They'll hear only the good stuff and sugar-coat the process, or focus exclusively on the bad stuff and jump on staff to fix the problems without delay.

Neither reaction is helpful. Instead, try to reinforce the positive, and offer calm, rational suggestions for dealing with the negative. Don't fall into the trap of becoming your loved one's "fixer." Whenever possible, it's best if they do this themselves. You're still your loved one's advocate, but she's the one who has to live in this setting, and she's got to learn how to deal with staff on her own.

Long-term adjustment

Resident and family alike tend to try to rush the process, but in most cases it's difficult to gauge the success of a move until your loved one has had several months in the new setting. Those with less experience in moving might not truly settle in until a year or more has passed. Keep in mind that events in the nursing home can slow the adjustment process. Changes in staff, the death of a roommate, the arrival of a disruptive neighbor, the onset of new medical problems—all these things make the settling-in period bumpier and longer than expected.

How can you tell when your loved one has made the transition from "settling in" to "long-term adjustment"? Look for several things:

- *Development of new routines.* When Mom starts to refer to her lunches with Mrs. Jones or her "date" with the physical therapist, it's a sign that she's beginning to see these things as routine parts of her new life.
- *Deepened ties to staff and residents.* When Dad voices concern about his favorite nurse's sprained wrist, or Mom wants to shop for a birthday gift for her roommate, you know these people have become important to your loved one.
- *Anticipation of upcoming events at the facility.* It often comes as a surprise to family when their socially isolated father starts looking forward to a trip or a party, but it's actually a pretty common reaction. As residents experience these events, they begin to enjoy them—even if they weren't the kinds of things they used to like.
- *Decreased dependence on you.* The day may come when your visit—once the center of Mom's day—pales next to the bridge tournament. She may even start to hint that you need a "vacation" from visiting. Don't be offended—she still needs you. It's just that she has a life of her own...again.

CONJUGAL VISITS

Not surprisingly, spouses separated by differing care needs want private time alone, for lovemaking, talking, or just being together. Facility staff will be glad to make the necessary arrangements. Most facilities have established procedures for conjugal visits ("Do Not Disturb" doorknob hangers, alternate arrangements for roommates, etc.), and they'll arrange things as discreetly as possible, given some advance notice. If your loved one needs special assistance from staff to prepare for conjugal visits (for example, securing a catheter), these matters can also be dealt with in advance. Don't be shy: Ask the social services director how such needs are handled at the facility.

Building New Routines in a Changing Relationship

Just as your loved one must work to build new structure into her life, you as a caregiver must work to build new routines into your changing relationship. The trick here is to find a set of routines that works for both of you—routines that keep you connected but still allow you to live independent lives.

For most people, regular contact with a nursing home resident comes through three sources: *visits, off-grounds trips,* and *telephone, mail, and e-mail contact.* Only you and your loved one can decide what balance is right for you.

Visits in the Nursing Home

Unlike hospitals, most nursing homes have liberal visiting hours. However, as you'll soon discover, each nursing home has its own unique rhythm, and residents' schedules tend to be quite full. Yes, your visit will usually get priority, but be prepared for a few glitches early on: If your arrival coincides with that of the physical therapist, you're going to find yourself cooling your heels until the therapy session is over. Until you get into the swing of things, you may feel as if you're forever showing up at an awkward moment.

The rhythm of the nursing home

Nursing homes have fairly regimented schedules. Residents must be washed, dressed, and ready for meals at specific times. (Many residents have to eat at a particular hour to accommodate a medication regimen.) Therapy sessions and group activities can be hard to reschedule on short notice. Outside consultants generally arrive during standard business hours; most off-grounds trips take place during the daytime as well.

To a surprising degree, the nursing home day is defined by the staff's shift changes, which usually take place at 7:00 A.M., 3:00 P.M., and 11:00 P.M. The half-hour periods right before and right after those times tend to be pretty hectic—people are arriving, leaving, and settling into their work routine. Shift changes can be difficult for some residents as well, especially those who are disoriented or confused.

Bedtime in nursing homes is earlier than you think. For many residents, bedtime rituals begin soon after the dinner dishes are cleared. Evenings tend to be quiet, although a few activities may be held quite late, to accommodate night-owls with disrupted sleep patterns. (Most of us sleep less as we age, and the average seventy-year-old sleeps only six hours per night.)

Timing of visits

New residents' schedules are established within the first day or two and fine-tuned as staff get to know the person better. Most facilities give residents printed copies of their schedules as soon as they're available, to help them adjust to the new routines. To time your visits correctly, learn the schedule. Figure out when your loved one will have some "down time." (Late mornings, late after-noons, and early evenings are good bets.) Whenever possible, avoid visiting when hard-to-reschedule events are taking place, like bathing or therapy.

During the initial settling-in period, it's best if you avoid interrupting activities that help the resident connect with new neighbors. You might enjoy meeting Mom's roommate, but don't let your presence distract from the roommate's account of her beagle's life story—this might be an important opportunity for the two of them to bond.

While some people delight in "surprising" their loved ones, the planned visit is usually far more appreciated by residents and staff. Residents like knowing when you'll be there, so they can look forward to your visit and plan around it. (Besides, the joke's on you if your arrival coincides with a roommate's enema.)

Length of visits

This should be determined by the resident's mood and attention span. If things seem to be going well, stay longer. If not, leave sooner. If you can't tell how things are going, err on the side of brevity. Shorter, more frequent visits tend to be better than fewer, longer ones, especially for confused or demented residents. If your schedule permits, you might find that popping in for a few minutes once or twice a day—perhaps on your way to and from work—is better than spending all day Sunday with your loved one.

It's easy to forget that when you're visiting, your loved one is your "host"—she might not feel comfortable telling you to leave. Don't wait for her to tell you she's tired or that your arrival coincided with her hairdressing appointment. Instead, watch carefully: She'll let you know in her own, subtle way. (Many people clam up or become a bit vague in their answers, hoping you'll take the hint and scram.)

THE GUEST WHO WOULDN'T LEAVE...

Every nursing home has at least one: the sibling, spouse, or child who arrives each day at lunchtime and stays until the final flicker of the latest late-night talk show. Staff and other residents get to know these honorary neighbors as well as any resident—whether they want to or not!

At first, these stalwart visitors' devotion is noted and praised. Soon, though, the grumbling starts (though usually when the visitor isn't around). If staff members begin to joke about "charging you rent," take the hint. They're trying to tell you as nicely as possible that you're overstaying your welcome.

Who should go?

Everyone who wants to visit should do so, but not all at once. While nursing homes almost always have parlors, gardens, and lounges available, many folks like to meet with visitors in "their" space. If your loved one has a private room, there's no problem. But if he's sharing a room with two other men, and they all have company at the same time, you'll soon reach standing-room-only capacity. If possible, spread visits out—you go one day, your brother goes the next day, and so on. Special occasions may warrant getting the whole gang together, but only if the resident can tolerate a crowd.

People sometimes wonder if children should visit loved ones in nursing homes. It depends on two things: the age of the child and the condition of the resident. Generally, infants and toddlers seem comfortable in nursing homes. Slightly older children may be frightened or confused by some of the sights and sounds. If your loved one's health and appearance have taken a significant turn for the worse, consider carefully whether it's appropriate for a young child to see him. Sometimes it's kinder to let children hang on to their memories of a healthy, vigorous grandparent rather than introducing them to harsh reality.

Older children who visited the resident at home can—and should—continue to visit after the resident moves to the facility, but they should hold off on visiting when they are ill. Nursing facilities almost always have some residents with impaired immune systems, and visitors with upper respiratory infections may be banned during flu season (more on this in Chapter 9).

ROOMMATE CONFLICTS

If you've ever watched *The Odd Couple* on TV, picture this: Felix and Oscar still living together, but now they're in their eighties, with health problems, and instead of sharing a spacious Park Avenue apartment, they're crammed into a single room. Not a pretty picture, is it?

Roommate conflicts are one of the most common problems in nursing homes, and can be among the hardest to address. Clashes over TV volume, bathroom habits, loved ones' use of shared space....you name it. Add cultural, religious, and ethnic differences, and it's a wonder two nursing home roommates *ever* get along. Roommates are generally assigned by nursing and/or social work staff, and in most settings changes can be made if the residents are truly miserable. The rule is usually that "the complainer moves," which makes sense, but keep in mind that moves within a nursing home often involve some cost and inconvenience (for example, telephone and cable services have to be relocated). If your loved one is transferred to a unit covered by a different physician, he might have to change doctors as well (along with nurses and other familiar staff). And there's no guarantee that the next roommate will be better than the last.

Of course, a private room would solve all these problems, but it's far more expensive than a shared one, and much harder to get, since most facilities reserve private rooms for residents whose medical needs require quarantine. It's wise to give your loved one some time to work out a roommate conflict before intervening too forcefully. Social work staff are often skilled in negotiating roommate truces and "ceasefires," as they face these situations pretty frequently.

Remember, too, that children tend to absorb a lot of visitor and staff attention. If your loved one is feeling a bit needy himself, he might not be happy about sharing the limelight with someone far cuter, even if he doesn't say so directly. Other residents sometimes resent the noise and activity children can generate. Some residents may become snippy around high-energy kids; other residents (especially confused ones) become agitated and fretful. Keep in mind that you are the visitor here: If your presence is upsetting other residents, you owe it to them to quiet things down or leave. Wouldn't you want others to do the same for your loved one?

ANIMALS IN THE NURSING HOME

Many nursing homes have resident birds and fish, which are housed in common areas and cared for by staff. Some facilities have dogs, cats, rabbits, or guinea pigs, but recurring concerns about infection control have made this practice less common in recent years. Most facilities do have regularly scheduled "pet visits" from local animal centers or volunteer agencies. Animal visitors are chosen for their quiet demeanor and obedience—unruly critters need not apply. Handlers are trained to be sensitive to residents' needs and are careful not to frighten phobic or confused residents. Most residents love these visits, and research has shown that animal guests yield a number of positive effects: They facilitate social interaction, lower blood pressure, elevate mood, and enhance residents' sense of well-being.

If you want to bring your own or your loved one's pet for a visit, check with the facility first. Most have leash rules, some have paperwork requirements, and a few ask for proof that the animal's vaccinations are current. Allocate extra time for visits when you bring a dog or cat along—you'll probably be a lot more popular than usual.

What should you do?

Pretty much what you'd do at home. If you used to spend time chatting or watching TV, just pick up where you left off. Eat lunch or dinner together. If you're not sure what to do, take this opportunity to develop some new common interests. Play chess or cards. Put a jigsaw puzzle together. Or try bird-watching in the garden, reading aloud, or strolling around the grounds—whatever feels comfortable.

Two activities bring with them special concerns. For both of these, think before you act:

- *Focusing on the past.* Reminiscing about the "good old days" can be a way of renewing longstanding bonds, but it can also deepen your loved one's sense of longing for things that once were but can never be again. If you know from experience that talking about your grandmother gets mother upset, don't do it unless it's absolutely necessary. On the other hand, if your mother finds joy in thinking about her mother, by all means, talk about her. (An important caveat: If your loved one is suffering from an advanced dementia, she may have difficulty separating past from present. This is generally not a problem for her, so try not to let it upset you. Correcting her errors isn't helpful—she's not going to "get it" no matter how hard you try. Just listen, nod, and gently steer the conversation elsewhere.)

• *Sharing bad news.* Your husband needs surgery, your daughter failed math, and on top of all that, the cat has worms. You might be tempted to shield your loved one from bad news, but unless there's a compelling reason to do so, it's better to be honest. You needn't dwell on troubles, but neither should you hide them. Admission to a nursing home shouldn't deprive people of the right to be involved in their loved ones' lives, in good times or bad. Besides, if you're sad or irritable over problems at work, your loved one might assume you're angry with her if you leave her in the dark.

WHAT'S FOR DINNER?

After roommate conflicts, the most common complaints among nursing home residents have to do with the food. It's too hot, too cold, too chewy, or too mushy; there's too much to eat or not enough. Sometimes residents' complaints reflect serious health issues (like improper food storage), but many complaints are really matters of taste ("Too spicy!"). If possible, try to sample a meal at some point. Visitors are often welcome to share in meals for a modest fee, though the dietary department requires advance notice. Eating nursing home food might sound like a distasteful proposition, but if you aren't willing to sample the fare, how can you insist that your loved one eat it?

The Off-Grounds Pass

You don't spend all your time in your home, and your loved one doesn't want to spend all his time in his. Off-grounds visits can be a highlight of the nursing home resident's day, so long as you use a bit of common sense. Go where you usually go—your home, friends' homes, church, the mall, museums—and do what you usually do. Get errands out of the way (banking and so forth), then reward yourselves by having fun.

Three guidelines can make your off-grounds visits go as smoothly as possible:

- *Don't forget about bathroom needs.* If your loved one has to use the bathroom frequently, or with little advance warning, avoid large, crowded areas where lines for the facilities tend to be long. If your loved one needs a wheelchair-accessible bathroom, locate the nearest one ahead of time. Find out if you need a key to access it and if so, where you go to get it.
- *Avoid the busiest times.* If your loved one is upset by crowds, schedule visits to popular stores and restaurants during "down" times. Ditto for banks and movie theatres.
- *Prepare for an early exit.* Your loved one may tire more easily than before, so be ready to cut a trip short if necessary. Some events (like concerts) can be hard to leave gracefully; other exits just take time—for example, crowded holiday malls. Don't be upset if your plans get disrupted. That's par for the course where an ill or aging family member is concerned.

Leaving and Returning: Practical Considerations

Oftentimes, the most difficult aspects of an off-grounds trip are the departure and return. A little advance planning can go a long way toward smoothing these transitions.

HOLIDAY GATHERINGS

For some nursing home residents, the prospect of missing an important family gathering can be devastating. However, many have trouble tolerating the noise and bustle that are a part of these festivities. If your loved one starts to fade during such an event, find her a quiet spot to relax. Let her rest in the den and put her feet up. Or ask a friend or relative to chat with her one-on-one. If she finds pets soothing, see if the dog could use some petting, or let her gaze at the fishtank.

Sign-outs

Except for those residing in secure units, nursing home residents are free to come and go as they please—with some restrictions. Your loved one is in a nursing home because of her medical needs, and the facility is legally responsible for her safety. Thus, a doctor's order is required for off-grounds passes. This usually takes the form of a "standing order" in the resident's chart, executed on request. Facilities ask that residents give advance notice if they won't be present for meals or therapies, so schedules may be altered accordingly. Some facilities allow residents to leave unescorted, while others insist that a "responsible party" (approved by the resident and/or her health care proxy) be present. You'll be asked to sign out when you leave, noting your departure time, intended destination, estimated return time, and phone numbers where you can be reached in an emergency. Visitors sometimes chafe at this, feeling that the facility is being nosy, but a formal sign-out is actually a legal requirement, designed to guard against kidnapping or wandering off. Overnight visits are allowed, but require extra preparation and sometimes generate a "bedhold" fee. Check with the nursing home in advance.

Equipment

If your loved one needs a wheelchair, portable oxygen tank, or other medical devices, make sure you know how to transport and operate the equipment before you leave the nursing home. Some tasks (like unfolding a collapsible walker) look easy, but they can be tricky if you've never done them before. Staff will be happy to teach you, but advance notice will be welcome (sometimes essential, if staff are busy). Check ahead of time to be sure your destination has an accessible entrance and parking area.

When confronted by an oxygen tank or heart monitor, it's easy to get distracted and neglect the simple stuff. A forgotten hearing aid or pair of reading glasses can ruin an otherwise wonderful trip. Try to make a mental list of these necessities, or a written list if you need one, and check to see that you have everything you need before you take off.

Medications

If your loved one is in a setting where staff administer medication, they will prepare packets of needed medication to take with you, along with instructions for proper administration. If a medication needs to be taken with food or liquid, they'll tell you. Pay attention, and ask questions until you're certain you understand the instructions. If necessary, write them down.

Getting out the door (and back in at the end)

Most folks adjust well to the leaving and returning routines you help them develop. However, the beginning and end of an off-grounds trip can be complicated by the resident's reluctance to leave or return. Many residents express their reluctance indirectly (for example, by not being dressed at the appointed time), and on occasion these problems can escalate into battles, particularly if the settling-in period has been bumpy, or the person's physical or mental condition is deteriorating.

You may be able to address this hurdle by enlisting the help of others. Staff can ensure that your loved one is booted up and ready to roll when you arrive, as long as you give them advance notice. A loved one who balks at going back when you raise the issue may be more cooperative with a friend. Calm, steadfast resolve is your best response to problems in this area, but if leaving and returning prove unmanageable despite your best efforts, consider putting off-grounds trips on hold for a while.

Staying Connected Between Visits

It is important to stay in contact with your loved one between visits, especially if you can't visit frequently. Most of us have a preferred mode of communication (mail, telephone, or e-mail). Letters and phone calls remain the most popular modes of communication among nursing home residents, but e-mail is becoming more popular every day.

Try to tailor your communications to your loved one's preferences. Provide family and friends with the resident's new contact information as soon as possible, and encourage them to call and write. You needn't wait for Christmas or Valentine's Day to call or send a note—the "thinking of you" message is always welcome (especially so because it's unexpected). If friends and family members are willing, have them call and write at different times, so the resident gets a steady flow of communication, rather than an avalanche of letters and phone calls all at once.

Telephone contact

In most facilities, staff will provide assistance in making phone calls if asked. Keep in mind that access to the public phone may be restricted during the busiest times, depending on how many others need to use the phone and which staff people are available to help. Prepaid phone cards that allow your loved one to make long-distance calls with less hassle make great gifts. If your loved one has private in-room phone service, help her set up "speed dial" options for frequently-called numbers. Private phones can also be equipped with sound enhancers for hearing-impaired residents. (Speaker phones should be avoided, though—they annoy other residents.)

Contact by mail

Be sure your loved one has an appropriate stock of notecards, stamps, and other materials—stationery and rolls of stamps make good gifts for the older person with an extensive correspondence list. A trip to the store to get holiday cards can be a good excuse for an outing (but buy stamps ahead of time—a long wait in line at the post office will put anyone in a bad mood). If the person has poor vision or shaky handwriting, consider volunteering your secretarial skills—it's a nice way to pass time during a visit. Type letters to the resident, and print

SENIOR SURFERS

Stereotypes notwithstanding, older adults are active Internet users. In fact, industry surveys indicate that Internet users aged fifty and over average more than eight hours per week online; more than a third purchased something over the Internet in the past year. Nearly 40 percent of people between fifty-five and sixty-five are regular Internet users, and almost 20 percent of those seventy-five or older go online at least once a week.

If your loved one needs some help getting started, perhaps you can share your knowledge. (It can sometimes be a fun "bonding" experience.) Or hook them up with *Seniornet*—a company created to provide computer and technology information (including Internet help) for seniors. They can be reached at 900 Lafayette Street, Suite 604, Santa Clara, CA 95050. (You can also contact them by phone at 408-615-0699 or online at www.seniornet.org.)

them in a large font. If you write letters by hand, take your time and make them neat. Many older folks have vision limitations that make reading messy handwriting almost impossible.

E-mail

E-mail is still a novelty to some nursing residents, although virtually all facilities offer Internet access and many older folks enjoy communicating by computer once they get the hang of it. Of course, some seniors find the whole concept of e-mail communication confusing and foreign. If your loved one falls into the latter group, ask e-mail–happy family members to send messages directly to you. You can either print out the messages or share these good tidings verbally during visits.

Establishing a communication routine

Late-night phone calls aren't much fun, so establish times when your loved one shouldn't call you, except in an emergency. But be considerate of your loved one's schedule, too—she might hesitate to set limits on you, so ask directly: When are the best times to call? When should I avoid calling? If roommates are involved, be considerate of them as well.

All routines, no matter how carefully constructed, get disrupted on occasion. Yours will too, and here's what to do:

- *Vacations.* Families sometimes feel guilty about going on vacation and leaving their loved one behind, and on occasion they'll deal with this guilt by not saying anything about the trip until they're halfway out the door. Don't do this. It's unkind, and you might be rewarded with a series of "emergency" calls from an angry care receiver who doesn't cope well with surprises. Under no circumstances should you leave home for more than a day without telling your loved one—she might get scared when she can't reach you. And be sure to inform the nursing home as well—it needs to know where to reach you in an emergency.
- *Business trips.* Advance notice is strongly recommended. If your job requires that you travel on short notice, designate an alternate contact person the facility can call in an emergency. This usually works better than leaving a list of phone numbers where the facility might—or might not—be able to reach you.

TAKE CARE OF YOURSELF

Now that your loved one has taken up residence in a nursing home, this is a good time to remind yourself of the key principles of caregiving. (It's easy to forget about these when things get hectic.) So take a few moments to review the framework for caregiving we described in Chapter 1, and if you're feeling overwhelmed, take action:

- *Find support at the facility.* Some nursing homes offer support groups for family members or can direct you to places that do.
- *Find support in the community.* Consider joining a community support group. (Check with local agencies on aging, or use the contact information at the back of the book.)
- *Seek spiritual support.* A trusted member of your church, synagogue, or mosque can help put things in perspective.

8

Confrontation or Partnership— It's Up to You: A Down-and-Dirty Guide to Nursing Home Politics

Helen looked around the room. She was surrounded by familiar faces. Her social worker was there, and her physical therapist as well. The activities director and the dietician were sitting side by side, talking quietly. At the head of the table was Anne, the information nurse—a take-charge woman who ran care plan meetings at Harter Hall. Anne was thumbing through papers, making notes here and there. Charts and folders were piled high on the table in front of her.

Anne looked up from her papers. She cleared her throat, and the room grew quiet. She put down her pen and began.

"OK, let's review. Helen joined us in February from Mayfair General, following a CVA with left hemiparesis. She's also treated for hypertension and diabetes, and she's waiting on cataract surgery. Since last review, March second, she's been in PT five times a week, OT three times a week. She had one fall, March eleventh—no injuries, no ill effects. No med changes. She's had a seven-pound weight gain, and Dr. Small has us monitoring her blood sugars BID."

Anne's voice softened as she turned to the two women sitting to her right. "Helen, Alice? Any questions so far?"

"No," said Helen. Alice shook her head.

Anne turned to her left. "Bill? An update?" Bill was Helen's physical therapist.

Bill paused for a moment, collected his thoughts. "Well," he said slowly, "Helen's balance has improved, and she's made good progress with the rolling walker. We've got to keep working on that left leg, though. We've got quite a ways to go there."

Anne made a note on the page in front of her. She gestured toward Helen's occupational therapist. "Helen, Jill says you're having trouble dressing?"

Helen exhaled slowly. "Yes," she said. "That's true. The shoes are OK, but I can't get my stockings right. I hate that stretcher-thing…I just can't get the hang of it."

Alice's eyebrows furrowed. A questioning look came over her face. Jill leaned over and put her hand on Alice's arm.

"It's an assistive device," she explained, "to help people with limited mobility dress on their own."

"Oh." Alice looked relieved. "Well, that's not really a problem, right? Since Mom's going to assisted living, I mean. There'll be someone there to help her get dressed, I thought."

"That's true," said Jill. "Still, we want her to be as independent as possible before discharge." Jill patted Alice's arm again, and settled back in her seat.

"All right, then," said Anne. "So where are we?"

There was a pause, then Bill spoke up. "The cataract surgery?"

"Mmm…tell you what," said Anne. "Why don't we hold off on that till we get a bead on Helen's OT and blood sugars. In the meantime, let's look at meds. Darlene? Where are we with these?"

Every nursing home has its own unique history, but in some ways all nursing homes are very much alike. To get things accomplished, you must work *with* the system, not against it. And to work with the system, you must understand it. You must learn each person's role within the institution and figure out which people are the "movers and shakers"—the people who can really help you get things done.

In this chapter, we discuss the different roles played by nursing home staff, the settings where you can lobby on your loved one's behalf, and effective strategies for getting things accomplished when you need to.

Nursing Home Staff: The Cast of Characters

Nursing homes must meet a wide variety of resident needs, from medical care and physical therapy to religious and social programming. It's not unusual for a large facility to have the equivalent of two hundred—even three hundred—full-time employees. Here's what they do.

Administrators

The *Nursing Home Director* makes decisions regarding finances, policy, and personnel. The Director is the bridge between the organization and various regulatory agencies, and must stay current on changes in Medicare and Medicaid laws, as well as federal and state rulings related to nursing home administration.

In smaller nursing homes, the Director is involved in the day-to-day life of the facility—you'll likely run into her when you visit. In larger facilities, the Director is rarely on-grounds. She spends most of her time managing business affairs, and delegates day-to-day responsibilities to various department heads. The largest nursing homes often have a separate *Chief Fiscal Officer* who focuses solely on financial issues.

Physicians

The *Medical Director* is a physician who makes medical policy decisions at the facility. In larger homes, the Medical Director serves primarily as supervisor and spokesperson for medical matters; in smaller homes, the Medical Director also carries his or her own patient caseload.

Each nursing home resident has an *attending physician* who makes decisions about the person's medical care and communicates these decisions to facility staff. Attending physicians are not employed by the facility but must be *privileged* or *credentialed* to provide services there. (Their professional credentials must be formally approved by a committee headed by the Medical Director.)

Family members often assume that nursing home residents are seen by the attending physician every day, but this is almost never the case. When a resident has an acute medical problem, the physician may see him weekly, but as things stabilize, visits become less frequent. In many states, physicians are required to

home patients once a month. A long-term resident with stable
ⁿ seen only once every sixty days.

Nursing staff

he attending physician is like an orchestra conductor, coordinating the
_ments of many different players. Among the most important players are
nbers of the nursing staff, who provide much of the day-to-day care. Nurs-
staff includes:

- *The Director of Nursing (DON).* The DON is a registered nurse
  who oversees all aspects of direct patient care. The DON is responsible for nursing care staffing—making sure there are an
  adequate number of hands on deck at all times. The DON also
  works to ensure smooth interactions among different members
  of the treatment team. In smaller facilities, the DON may be a
  hands-on caregiver; in larger nursing homes, the DON's admin-
  istrative duties are a full-time job.
- *Review staff.* Most facilities have specially trained nurses who
  keep track of residents' Medicare status and make sure that
  charts and care plans meet federal and state standards. Review
  staff provide little hands-on care, but they are an integral part of
  the treatment team, taking part in care planning meetings and

CAN THE RESIDENT CONTINUE WITH HER DOCTOR AFTER ADMISSION?

Although a physician's nursing home visits are covered by Medicare, Medicaid, and other insurance sources, these visits are usually reimbursed at a
lower rate than standard office visits. Physicians are not paid for travel time,
paperwork, or time needed to answer the complex care questions many
nursing home patients generate. Because of this, many physicians choose
not to seek nursing home privileges, and your loved one may have to change
doctors when she enters the facility. Check with your doctor on this ahead
of time.

freeing direct care staff from some of the more onerous paper-work requirements. Some aspects of care that require extra training and very precise charting may be addressed by *nurse spe-cialists* (for example, *a wound care nurse*), who provide service and document progress only within their area of expertise.

- *The charge nurse.* Every shift has a *charge nurse*, who supervises care staff on duty during that shift. The charge nurse tracks changes in a resident's condition (including injuries or illnesses) and informs the resident's physician as needed. She also informs the resident's family of health changes, new orders, and new consultation requests.

- *Line staff.* Most complex nursing tasks (such as starting IV lines and placing catheters) are performed by *registered nurses (RNs)*, who hold college degrees in nursing. *Licensed practical nurses (LPNs)* undergo briefer training and may perform certain tasks only under supervision of a registered nurse. Basic care tasks—bathing, toileting, grooming, etc.—are handled by *certified nursing assistants* ("aides").

Social services

The *Director of Social Services* ensures that the resident's social and emo-tional needs are met. This includes everything from ensuring that residents have sufficient underwear to helping someone apply for Medicaid. The Director of Social Services compiles the initial social history for each resident, makes sure that advance directives and other legal documents are in place, and monitors each resident's adjustment to the facility. Special services related to patients' emotional needs (for example, psychotherapy from an outside provider) are co-ordinated by the Social Service director.

Dietary services

The *Director of Dietary Services* is usually a registered dietician with train-ing in the nutritional needs of elderly and ill patients. The Director works in concert with the *Dietary Chief*, who runs the kitchen, supervises staff, orders food and supplies, and helps implement diets for residents with special needs (for example, diabetic diets). Dietary staff who serve as "feeders" consult with

---

THE WORLD OF THE AIDE

Being an aide in a nursing home is among the most challenging jobs on earth. During a typical eight-hour shift, an aide may bathe, toilet, dress, and feed as many as fifty or sixty people. Many residents are not particularly receptive to being helped, and they may curse, bite, hit, spit…you name it.

As if that isn't enough, every patient contact must be documented in writing, and the aide may not leave until documentation is complete, even if his shift is over. The pay is poor, the hours unpredictable, and if there's a problem, supervisory staff usually side with the resident and the resident's irate family members.

Is it any wonder that in most nursing homes, aide turnover is high? Try to be understanding, and treat aides with respect. It's the right thing to do, and besides, when aides are happier, residents get better care.

---

speech therapists and nursing staff to learn how to work with residents who have chewing problems, swallowing problems, or other food-related difficulties.

Activities services

The *Activities Director* ensures that each resident has an activity schedule tailored to his or her needs, and keeps track of the resident's participation in this schedule. Members of the activity staff plan social programs for the nursing home, compose "events calendars," organize off-grounds trips, arrange celebrations for various occasions, and generally ensure that there's little "down time" in the life of the residents. Activities staff visit room-bound residents individually and plan on-unit events for those with mobility limitations.

Pastoral/Clergy

Some nursing homes have in-house clergy on staff, who address residents' spiritual needs. The resident pastor conducts services in his or her denomination and works with clergy from other religious groups to ensure that all residents have access to religious services and spiritual guidance. In nursing homes without in-house clergy, social service staff are responsible for seeing that residents' spiritual needs are met; outside clergy are brought in to perform religious services and other functions.

Therapies and ancillary services

Rehabilitation Services staff are usually independent contractors, not employees of the facility. Here's what they do:

- *Physical therapists* have expertise in restoring physical function. Locomotion is the most frequent issue here, as many residents must learn to walk again following a hip fracture or stroke. Physical therapists also help enhance strength, balance, and coordination, and are occasionally called upon to deal with more subtle muscle control issues, such as teaching Kegel exercises for bladder control.
- *Occupational therapists (OTs)* help residents recover lost ADLs (dressing, bathing, etc.). Many OTs also do *home evaluations*: They go to the resident's home, assess the environment, and suggest assistive devices that would make the home safer (for example, grab bars in the bathroom). On occasion, an OT will advise against discharge if they feel that someone won't be able to function safely in the home.
- *Speech and language therapists* help patients enhance their language processing skills. Speech therapists are also involved in treating *dysphagia* (chewing and swallowing problems), and work closely with dietary staff to develop proper diets and feeding strategies for dysphagic residents.

Housekeeping and maintenance

Housekeeping staff make beds, change linens, do laundry, clean bathrooms, beds, and floors, and use established procedures to dispose of trash properly. The director of housekeeping services also makes sure the facility complies with federal and state guidelines regarding sanitation and infection control. Because most nursing homes house incontinent residents and those with contagious illnesses, this can be quite a challenge.

Maintenance staff keep the physical plant in working order. They maintain the heating, cooling, plumbing, electric, and emergency alert systems; mow grass; clear snow; and keep the grounds litter-free. They also maintain the medical equipment and major appliances. The maintenance crew usually help new residents move in, and they're the first ones called when a car won't start, a hearing aid battery jams, or a walker wheel begins to squeak.

Allied and support services

Few nursing homes have a full complement of specialists on the payroll— it's just too expensive. Instead, most facilities contract with independent providers for specialty services. The most common specialty providers are dentists, ophthalmologists, psychologists, psychiatrists, podiatrists, radiologists (who have mobile units for on-site screening), phlebotomists (who draw blood for testing), and ambulance service personnel (who transport frail or bedfast patients to and from the facility).

Admissions, billing, and human resources

These are the paperwork folks, who make sure forms are filled out, bills submitted, and fees collected. Admissions staff make sure that required documents are in place when a resident is admitted, transferred, or discharged. Billing staff keep track of Medicare, Medicaid, and secondary insurance paperwork. Larger homes may have a separate human resources department, which coordinates wages and benefits, helps recruit and retain staff, and organizes facility-wide safety training sessions. Some larger nursing homes also have staff-education specialists, who ensure that all employees are properly trained in the laws, policies, and procedures related to their work in the facility.

Interfacing with Staff: Your Arenas of Influence

Family members usually have lots of questions about their loved one's treatment—and quite a few opinions as well. Nursing home staff will welcome this input, as long as it is expressed appropriately. You'll have opportunities to ask questions and voice your opinions in several different settings.

Admission review meetings:
Where plans are formed

From the moment your loved one enters a skilled nursing facility, everyone works together to help her resume the highest possible level of independent living. Discharge planning begins on the day of admission, and the first step in discharge planning is assessment. The new nursing home resident goes through what may seem like an endless stream of exams and interviews—physical exams, social histories, dietary evaluations, and so forth. Sometimes it feels as though the assessments will never end.

But end they do, and within a few days of admission, members of the treatment team assemble in a formal *admission review meeting* and outline the initial *care plan*—the "blueprint" of therapies designed to help residents achieve their treatment goals. Care plan goals are very specific and include precise, measurable outcomes that the resident must meet before moving forward. Treatments are also described precisely—what gets done, who does it, how frequently, and how long.

Residents and family members are invited to the admission review meeting, but not all families choose to go. If you can find some way to attend this important first gathering of the treatment team, do. First impressions are important, and this is your chance to show the staff that you intend to stay involved in your loved one's treatment.

Care plan meetings:
Where decisions are made

Goals and treatments outlined in the initial care plan are usually reassessed every two or three weeks in acute rehab settings. In long-term care, a *care plan review meeting* is held once every three months (more often if there's a change in the resident's condition) to discuss progress and see what challenges remain. Residents and family members are encouraged to attend care plan meetings so they can share their observations, ask questions, and make suggestions. These are the arenas where future care plans (including discharge plans) are discussed, so listen carefully: Staff will tell you what your loved one can realistically expect to achieve as things progress.

You might not be able to attend every care plan meeting, but you should try to attend them periodically (at least every other meeting, if possible). Let staff know ahead of time if you plan to attend—they'll put your loved one's review in a convenient spot on the agenda when they know you're going to be there.

Resident and family councils: Where concerns are voiced

Most nursing homes have *resident councils*—formal meetings (usually monthly) in which residents share their experiences and make suggestions for improving the facility. Social services staff help organize these meetings and see that representatives from the major treatment disciplines are available to address residents' questions or concerns.

Many nursing homes also have *family councils*, which focus on the concerns of families and visitors. Try to attend these so you can stay abreast of goings-on at the facility. While nursing homes are under no legal obligation to respond to the councils' requests, most try to do so. Family council meetings can be an important arena of influence for the concerned family member.

CARE PLAN MEETINGS AND THE FUNDING DILEMMA

Care plan meetings are not only important from a treatment perspective, but they also help determine funding for future services. Funding sources, including Medicare, are usually quite flexible with respect to care plan "tweaking," as long as the resident is progressing toward his or her treatment goals. However, if a resident shows little or no improvement, this can turn into a problem—a big problem—down the line. When progress is slow, staff will try to motivate the resident as best they can. Continued failure to improve can result in loss of funding.

Here, then, is another good reason to attend care plan meetings: You'll stay up-to-date on progress and problems, have a chance to make suggestions when things aren't going well, and avoid an unpleasant surprise in the form of a Medicare turndown based on "insufficient progress" toward treatment goals.

Interactions with caregivers:
Where family and staff connect

If you spend time at the facility, you'll have plenty of opportunities to see staff in action and interact with them informally. A tremendous amount of in formation is shared in this manner, and many family members feel that it's actually the best means of communicating with staff and connecting with those who work with their loved one. Caregivers are human—they're more likely to take seriously concerns voiced by people they know, and the better they like you, the harder they'll work to meet your loved one's needs. You don't want to be a bother (don't turn into "The Guest Who Wouldn't Leave"), but do make an effort to get to know facility staff on an informal basis. A small investment of your time can pay great dividends in the long run.

THE LANGUAGE BARRIER

In many urban and suburban nursing homes, the majority of aides are people whose native tongue is not English. This can present a problem for residents who are confused or hearing-impaired, because the aide's strong accent may make communication difficult. Try to handle such situations with tact and kindness. Speak to the nursing supervisor if the language barrier is interfering with your loved one's care, but don't blame the aide. And if the aide is doing a good job in other areas, it may be best to tolerate a few communication glitches. (These should decrease over time, as aide and resident get to know each other better.)

Sadly, prejudice is often an issue when people from different backgrounds come together, as happens in most urban and suburban nursing homes. If your loved one isn't comfortable around people from different ethnic and racial groups, the likelihood of friction and miscommunication increases. If your loved one has led a somewhat isolated existence, you may want to give her a quick lesson in politically correct language, to diminish the likelihood that an unintended insult will slip out. Many nursing homes today address resident-staff interaction issues proactively, offering classes on cultural sensitivity for both residents and staff, and involving everyone in the celebration of holidays from a variety of cultures.

IS TIPPING ALLOWED?

Most facilities have stringent "no tipping" policies to ensure that all residents receive equal treatment. In reality, behind-the-scenes tipping does occur, creating some awkward situations for residents. No matter how grateful you feel toward a particularly helpful staff person, keep in mind that accepting money from residents or family members is usually grounds for being fired. If discovered, your generous impulse could cost this person her job. (Gifts to staff can also be tricky, although there is usually a little more leeway here, especially around the holidays.)

If you really want to reward staff, put your feelings in writing: Send a letter (or e-mail) to the nursing home administrator describing the wonderful things a particular staff member has done for your loved one. These kudos are taken into consideration when promotions are made, so they really do generate meaningful rewards for the nurse or aide who goes the extra mile.

Constructive Interventions: How to Get What You Want (and Be Loved While You're Doing It)

As the saying goes, you can catch more flies with honey than with vinegar. When interacting with nursing home staff, treat people as you would want them to treat you. The following strategies are most likely to produce the desired results.

- *Learn who does what—and why they do it.* All too often, harried family members grab the first staff person they see and insist that this person address some pressing need. The podiatrist gets told Mother's bedclothes are soiled; the aide gets quizzed about medication schedules. When communications are misdirected in this way, family members may get the impression that "nobody knows what's going on." Staff, in turn, feel like gofers—always being asked to track someone down or relay a message. Take time to learn who's who and what they do. Try to direct your questions to the right people. It facilitates communication and shows staff you care enough to put forth the extra effort.

• *Work with—not against—the facility's routines.* Coordinating the movements of many different people isn't easy and always involves compromise. Meals are scheduled earlier or later than you'd expect. Therapies take place when therapists can be there—sometimes at unusual hours. Meetings happen when the key players can attend, and at times that might conflict with your work or child-care responsibilities. Once staff know your scheduling constraints, they'll do their best to accommodate, but some flexibility on your part will be essential here.

• *Help staff understand the care receiver.* You've known your loved one a long time, and you've learned things about him that no one else knows. When you share this information with staff, everyone benefits. If Dad has a temper and tends to hit or kick when frustrated, let staff know this before someone finds out the hard way. If Mom gets moody without her before-dinner drink, tell everyone beforehand so they'll be prepared. Try not to let embarrassment prevent you from being honest about your loved one. You won't shock the nurses—they've heard it all before.

• *Back up the staff when a conflict occurs.* Don't get drawn into your loved one's private battles, if you can avoid it. It's better if they learn to hash these out themselves, and entering the fray can put you in an awkward position: Your loved one will expect you to take his or her side without question and will see you as a traitor if you don't. If you must get involved, keep an open mind. Listen to both sides, and when in doubt, back the staff. This will pay off down the line, when you need their support. Plus, an allied front is often the best way—sometimes the only way—to motivate a reluctant resident.

• *Express displeasure appropriately.* Be tactful and calm when communicating dissatisfaction. Don't gang up; instead, appoint one family member to act as spokesperson. Begin with the staff person most closely involved, then move up the "chain of command" until you get the result you want. Be as specific as possible (vague references to "poor care" rarely produce the de-

DESTRUCTIVE INTERVENTIONS: HOW *NOT* TO GET WHAT YOU WANT (AND MAKE ENEMIES IN THE PROCESS)

In stressful situations, family members often intervene in ways that make matters worse, not better. Several approaches are almost guaranteed to fail. These include:

- *Losing your temper.* No one likes being yelled at, and nursing home staff—who take abuse from residents on a regular basis—are not easily intimidated. If you feel yourself losing control over a problem in the nursing home, take "time out" until you regain control.
- *Threatening.* Like yelling, threatening will rarely produce the desired results. If you believe that your loved one is at risk or that a regulation is being violated, state your concerns clearly and calmly, and request a plan of action to address them. If you are not satisfied with the outcome after you have gone through the proper channels, advise the home's administrator that you intend to make a formal complaint—but don't say this unless you intend to follow through.
- *Ambushing staff.* How do you feel when a colleague or client grabs you on your way to an appointment, insisting that you drop what you're doing and deal with their problem right now—this very minute? If you find this frustrating, you can bet nursing home staff will, too. So don't do it.
- *Insisting on doing things your way.* Nursing home staff usually have tried-and-true strategies for dealing with problems—preferred approaches that have worked in the past. They may welcome your questions and suggestions, but they won't appreciate being lectured, or told that you have a "better" approach. Trying to "pull rank" on staff won't work well either—don't insist you know better because you have a higher degree than they do.

sired response), and provide concrete examples to illustrate the problem. Note dates, times, locations, people who were present—anything that strengthens your argument. And if, after doing all these things, you are still not satisfied, consider filing a formal complaint regarding your loved one's treatment.

REALITY BITES

Sad to say, there are some universal problems associated with nursing home life, including long wait times for call-bell response, items damaged or lost in the laundry, noisy neighbors, bad smells, and cranky, overworked staff. At some point, no matter how good the facility or how much you pay, you're going to encounter some of these problems. Bathroom assistance on a thirty bed unit covered by a single aide whose colleagues all called off on a stormy night is not going to be flawless, and she is likely to be quite harried (talk about your thankless jobs...).

While aggravating, these incidents usually result in embarrassment, inconvenience, and hurt feelings rather than serious injury, so before you bark at a staff person whose performance is less than perfect, remember that she doesn't control staffing patterns and has no way of magically summoning more help. You don't have to grin and bear bad service in silence, but a good general rule is to choose your battles carefully: Ignore rare glitches and one-time slipups and focus instead on chronic problems. Work your way through the chain of command to the appropriate administrator, and if necessary use family and resident councils for "strength in numbers."

When Complaining Is the Only Way

Every geographic region has at least one *Long-Term-Care Ombudsman*—a person who mediates disputes and disagreements that arise between nursing facilities and residents, or residents' families. When a complaint is filed, the ombudsman investigates and works with the facility to address the problem. If the ombudsman feels that further intervention is warranted, she notifies state and federal agencies, which then take action to protect the residents.

To avoid conflicts of interest, ombudsmen are not employees of the nursing home. Their services are paid for by the federal government, with funds channeled through each state's agency on aging. You pay nothing. The ombudsman's phone number must be posted in public areas at the facility, and it's usually included in the written materials that residents and families receive upon admission. You can also obtain contact information for an ombudsman from your local agency on aging. (Check the *Human Services* section of your phone book.)

As you might guess, facilities do not like being contacted by ombudsmen (or worse, state and federal investigators). By law, facilities cannot discriminate against residents who complain, but the reality is, a formal complaint often results in a permanent rift between staff and resident   particularly if staff feel they were not given an opportunity to address the problem in-house first. (See pages 149–150 for tips regarding this process.)

If your loved one's health is at stake, you've stated your concerns clearly, and they are not being addressed, then you really have no choice: You *must* proceed to a higher level. But it's best to think of a formal complaint as a "big stick"—don't swing it unless you have to. Don't alienate staff who are genuinely trying to meet your loved one's needs, and don't threaten staff as a way of controlling or intimidating them. Take it from us: They will not respond positively.

If you decide to take your dispute to an ombudsman, use the same strategy you would when making any sort of complaint:

- *Be specific* (give as much detail as possible)
- *Be accurate* (don't overstate your case to "get action")
- *Document the problem* (written descriptions, notes from conversations, photographs, etc.)
- *Link your complaint to an established legal right* (residents have many, families have few, and all are discussed in the following sections)

Legal rights of residents

Nursing home residents have a number of legal rights, ensured by federal and state regulations. These include:

- *Privacy.* Nursing home residents have the right to privacy for personal matters, and the right to "information privacy" as well: Staff and consultants may not disclose information about a resident, including the fact that they *are* a resident, unless they've been given permission to do so. Residents can also forbid staff from sharing information with specific people. ("If my brother John calls, do not give him any information about me.")

- *Dignity.* Nursing home residents have the right to be treated with dignity and respect — to be addressed politely, dressed appropriately, and handled gently when physical contact is required.

PHYSICAL AND CHEMICAL RESTRAINTS

By law, restraints of any kind are rarely used in nursing homes, except as a last resort—when a resident is so agitated that she is clearly a danger to herself. In such situations, two types of restraints may be used. *Physical restraints* are implements (like rear-fastening belts) that can be used to secure a resident to a bed or "Gerichair" (a sort of reclining chair on wheels for residents who can't use a wheelchair because of postural problems or agitation). *Chemical restraints* are drugs (for example, tranquilizers) used to calm an agitated resident. Physical and chemical restraints are used only when ordered by a physician, and the restrained resident must be monitored closely. Efforts must be made to find less restrictive treatments.

- *Money.* Nursing home residents have the right to manage their own money or to designate someone to do this for them. Residents also have the right to request that fees be outlined in writing before they receive a service.
- *Protection from abuse and exploitation.* Nursing home residents have the right to be protected from physical, sexual, emotional, and financial abuse and exploitation. (We discussed this issue in Chapter 3.)
- *Self-determination and autonomy regarding care decisions.* Nursing home residents (or those they appoint to make health care decisions for them) have the right to be informed regarding their medical condition and any treatments prescribed for them, including medications. They have the right to choose their own

doctor and to refuse treatments or consultations to which they object (with some restrictions). They also have the right to complain about care decisions and to demand resolution of grievances without reprisal.

- *Least restrictive alternative.* Nursing home residents have the right to as much physical freedom as possible, given their circumstances. Any physical or chemical restraints used must be medically necessary, properly ordered, documented, and monitored. It is inappropriate to restrain a resident or house that person in a locked unit, unless failure to do so would consitute a danger to the health and well-being of the resident or those around him.

- *Freedom of association.* Residents may interact with whomever they please. They also have a limited right to refuse to associate. (They may not refuse all human contact, but they need not take part in organized activities.) Residents can refuse visitors and can ask that specific people be denied access to them. While they cannot refuse to have a roommate, they do have the right to be informed of roommate changes in advance. Resident spouses have the right to share a room, unless it's medically contraindicated (and counterintuitive though it may seem, spouses also have the right to refuse to share a room if they wish to live separately).

WHEN FAMILY AND RESIDENT RIGHTS CONFLICT

When push comes to shove, the rights of a legally competent resident override those of his or her family. Thus, a competent resident can choose to withhold information about his condition or treatment from family members and can insist that staff do the same. Most residents don't do this, but they have the right to if they choose.

The bottom line: The resident's rights to privacy and self-determination "trump" the family's desire to be informed and involved—a frustrating situation, but understandable from a legal standpoint.

- *Freedom of religious, political, and sexual practices.* Unless a resident's behavior infringes on the rights of others, he has the right to practice his religion, express his political views, and engage in (private) sexual practices as he sees fit

Legal rights of family members

Family members do not have federally ensured legal rights in the same sense that residents do. Nonetheless, within the nursing home community, there are certain norms regarding what families can and cannot do. Here are the "rights" you should expect to have:

- *The right to be kept informed.* Family members should be informed of care plan changes. They should be informed immediately of significant changes in their loved one's health or functioning (for example, an injury or illness). Family members should also be informed when consultations are ordered, when insurance glitches arise, and when the resident is transferred to or from the facility, or moved from one part of the facility to another.
- *The right to challenge a care plan decision.* Family members have the right to ask questions about care plans until they are satisfied that they understand them. They also have the right to challenge a care plan decision, though unless the family member is the residents's durable power of attorney for health care, the final decision rests with the resident, the attending physician, and other members of the medical staff.
- *The right to be treated with dignity and respect.* Just as a nursing home resident has the right to be treated with dignity and respect, so do you. Family members should not be made to feel that they are unwanted or "in the way" (except, of course, during a crisis situation when staff must devote full attention to the resident).

WHO YOU GONNA CALL?

Knowing who to turn to can be challenging in a nursing home. If a resident has an urgent need, the answer's easy: Ring the call bell. When the problem is less pressing, ask the charge nurse, or go straight to the source:

Problem or Question	*Resource Person*
Questions about a treatment or medication	Attending Physician
Questions about an outside consultation	Attending Physician (who may refer you to the consultant)
Medical test results	Attending Physician
Progress in use of walker or wheelchair	Physical Therapist
Progress in use of assistive devices	Occupational Therapist
Speech or swallowing difficulties	Speech Therapist
Questions about diet or weight	Dietary Service Chief
Questions about change in health status	Charge Nurse
Reporting a fall or injury	Charge Nurse
Room change requests	Charge Nurse (who will consult with Social Service staff)
Roommate conflicts	Social Services
Privacy for private matters	Charge Nurse (if it's a one-time need) or Social Services (to have it regularly scheduled)
Help with Medicare or Medicaid paperwork	Social Services
Questions about billing	Financial Department

Problem or Question	Resource Person
Lost or damaged laundry	Housekeeping
Soiled bedding	Aide
Unsanitary bathroom/no paper products	Housekeeping
Problems with heat or air conditioning	Nursing staff (they'll contact Maintenance)
Equipment problems (stuck bed, etc.)	Aide
Activity scheduling problem/conflict	Activities Director
Spiritual guidance	Pastor/Clergy (if one is in-house), or Social Services
Questions about facility policies	Administrators
Suspected resident abuse	Charge Nurse
Complaints about care	Work up the ladder: 1) Aide 2) Charge Nurse 3) Director of Nursing 4) Attending Physician 5) Medical Director/ Other Administrator 6) Long-Term-Care Ombudsman
Complaint about a specific department	Work up the ladder: 1) Department Director 2) Administrator 3) Medical Director 4) Long-Term-Care Ombudsman

9

Old Age Ain't for Sissies: Late-Life Medical Problems and How to Deal with Them

I always show up at the same time each day —four o'clock during the week, noon on weekends. Doris seems comforted by a predictable schedule, and to tell you the truth, I like it, too. We're both creatures of habit, Doris and me. I guess that's why we've managed to stay together all these years.

Most days, things look pretty much the same when I arrive. Same staff on duty, same visitors, same residents in their usual spots. I like that, too—the sameness of it all. So you can imagine how surprised I was last Wednesday. I showed up at my usual time, but there were no residents in the common area. Warning signs were posted—everywhere, it seemed—and the staff seemed tense and moody. I waved, called out like I always do, but didn't get my usual greetings in return. Just a grim, forced smile and shake of the head from Roger, the charge nurse.

I started down the hall toward Doris's room, but Arlene— Roger's second-in-command—came up alongside me. I felt a gentle tug on my arm.

"Mr. Earle," she said quietly, "Come with me just a moment?"

She led me to a spot near the nurses' station, out of the line of traffic.

"Mr. Earle, we've got a flu bug going around in here. It might be best if you didn't visit with Doris today."

My heart skipped a beat. "Doris has the flu?" I imagined her in bed—scared, confused, now feverish and sick as well.

"No, Mr. Earle. Doris hasn't gotten it, thank goodness. But it's such a nasty strain this year, we're trying to do everything we can to keep it from spreading any further."

"Well," I said, "I can certainly understand that. The last thing you need is everyone throwing up at the same time. What a mess..."

"Yes, well, it's more serious than that, really. Flu in older folks is more than just nausea. People with weak immune systems are at serious risk."

"Really? I had no idea."

"Yes. We've already had to send three residents to the ER, and they're starting to turn people away. I don't know what we're going to do if this really takes off."

"My God. I didn't realize."

"Of course not. How would you know? Anyway, Doris is fine—she's OK so far—but I wanted to catch you before you headed in. If you've had any upper respiratory symptoms in the past week or so—any at all—it's probably best if you wait this out."

I didn't know what to say. Arlene patted my arm and smiled.

"It's up to you, Mr. Earle. If you want to go in, I can't stop you. And I know Doris would miss seeing you. Your visits are the highlight of her day. But think about it, all right? Just try to weigh whether some missed visits might be worth it if it can keep Doris from getting this god-awful bug."

I nodded but said nothing.

"Think about it, OK? Let me know what you decide." And with that, Arlene headed back toward the nurses' station. Another set of vistors had just arrived.

Old age ain't for sissies. The aging body doesn't work as well as it used to, and we become vulnerable in ways we could never have imagined. Illnesses like the flu, which might have been trivial just a few years earlier, can escalate into serious—even life-threatening—situations. A minor injury, like a broken wrist, may require weeks—maybe months—of rehab.

You don't have to be a doctor to be a good caregiver, but you do need to know enough about late-life health problems to help your loved one make sound treatment decisions. And if, at some point, you become your loved one's durable power of attorney for health care, you'll have to make these decisions on your own, with little or no input from the person whose health is at stake.

In this chapter, we provide basic information on late-life health problems and their treatment. We discuss the aging body, common medical problems in older adults, and the kinds of information you'll need to make sound treatment decisions with (or for) your loved one.

The Aging Body: Different Parts Work at Different Speeds

To understand health and illness in older adults, you must understand how human bodies change in later life. Every aging body is different, but a few principles hold true for most of us.

Some processes slow as we age

This is what we expect—to slow as we grow older. It's not true of everything, as we'll see shortly, but among the processes that slow in later life are:

- *Digestion and metabolism.* Over time, the body becomes less efficient in processing food, which takes longer to pass through the system, so more is absorbed. In addition, our *metabolism* (the rate at which we burn energy) usually slows with age, and excess weight becomes harder to shed.
- *Retrieval and reaction times.* Most people's cognitive skills (including memory) don't begin to decline until relatively late in

life. We do become less efficient at retrieving information from memory, however. (The information is still there—it just takes longer to find it.) Reaction time slows as well: We take longer to respond to new stimuli sights (like moving objects), sounds (like alarms), and so forth.

- *Recovery from injury or illness.* A lifetime of fighting off illness provides the immune system with a veritable fortress of *anti-bodies* (disease-fighting cells). As a result, we get better at fending off illness before it starts. The downside is, the aging immune system works less efficiently *after* we become ill. Healing takes longer, and sometimes older adults never recover fully from an illness (like the flu) that might have been trivial just a few years earlier.

- *Cell regeneration.* In most parts of the body, new cells are con-

---

TOO MUCH OF A GOOD THING?

Decades of society-wide antibiotic misuse have created serious problems in the nursing home. When people pressure their physicians to prescribe antibiotics for minor illnesses like colds, and then discontinue the prescription prematurely, before all the disease-causing organisms have been eradicated, the organisms mutate into resistant strains of "super-bugs." People need increasingly powerful medications to fight off invaders, and even those residents who used antibiotics properly may be unknowingly exposed to antibiotic-resistant microbes. The worst case-scenario: A *MRSA (Methicillin Resistant Staphylococcus Aureus)* infection makes its way through the nursing home, killing a number of residents in the process.

If your loved one contracts an antibiotic-resistant infection, he'll be quarantined. Warnings will be posted outside his room, advising you to contact nursing staff before entry. Staff will instruct you regarding precautions you should take before entering and leaving (for example, wearing a surgical mask and gloves, washing with disinfectant soap). Take these instructions seriously, and follow them precisely. If you don't, you'll place yourself at risk for a MRSA infection, and you could transmit the infection to vulnerable others, like children.

tinuously being produced to replace aging, dying cells. Skin, bone, muscle and blood cells still regenerate in later life but less quickly now than they once did. Because of this, skin becomes vulnerable to infection. Bones lose mass and become brittle, especially in women. When fractures occur, they heal less quickly and less completely.

Some processes accelerate as we age

It doesn't square well with our stereotypes, but some processes actually accelerate with age. These include:

- *Medication impact.* Because the kidneys work less efficiently in later life, it takes longer to rid the body of medication and its by-products. Drugs remain in the bloodstream longer, so dosages must be reduced. Most physicians modify prescriptions to take this into account, but over-the-counter medications, with their "one size fits all" dosages, remain problematic. The possibility of a dangerous drug interaction is higher now than it once was. And remember that alcohol, like other drugs, is metabolized less efficiently with age, so a given amount of alcohol may affect an older person more strongly than a younger one.

- *Spread of infection within the body.* Once an infection has entered the body of an older adult, it tends to spread quickly. Diseases can take over in a relatively short time, and because they stick around longer as well, the risk of serious complications, such as spread of disease to multiple organ systems, increases.

- *Organ deterioration.* After decades of use, many organs begin to wear down. The heart pumps less efficiently, the lungs extract less oxygen per breath, and the liver doesn't remove toxins as well as it used to. The body's organs are like machines: You can prolong their working life with good care, but nothing lasts forever.

Some things never change

Some things slow down, others speed up, and a few stay pretty much the same:

- *Underlying processes.* While certain processes slow down or speed up over time, the basic biological mechanics of life don't change. Breathing, eating, sleeping, regulating temperature—all these things occur the same way at age ninety as they did at age twenty.
- *Sense of self (Hello? It's still me in here....).* Because the body changes slowly, most older people maintain what psychologists call *constancy of experience*—they still feel like "their old selves" unless something drastic occurs (like loss of a limb). Our sense of self doesn't change much with age, and many older people carry around a mental image of themselves as younger and more vigorous than they really are. (Well, let's face it...most people in their thirties and forties do the exact same thing!)

Common Medical Problems in Older Adults

The sheer number of health problems that onset late in life can be intimidating to caregivers. Even if your loved one enjoyed decades of good health, don't be surprised if problems begin to accumulate as he moves into his seventies and beyond. And don't lose hope if your loved one develops multiple medical problems all at once: Nursing home staff have experience in dealing with challenging cases, and this won't be the first time they've seen someone with a complex pattern of illnesses.

In the following sections, we discuss major medical problems that afflict nursing home residents, along with treatments used to manage these illnesses and minimize their negative effects.

WHEN TO VISIT (AND WHEN TO WAIT)

Like Mr. Earle, well-meaning family members sometimes find themselves in a dilemma: Should they go ahead and visit even if they're sick or cancel the trip and disappoint their loved one? This is an issue you'll have to resolve on your own, and it really is up to you—staff can't prevent you from visiting if you want to. Here are some guidelines to help you decide:

- *Err on the side of caution.* If you think you're coming down with something, hold off on visiting, especially if your loved one's immune system is compromised. Be especially careful during outbreaks of flu and other illnesses in the nursing home—the last thing a sick resident needs is a second illness to battle at the same time.
- *Be especially careful with kids.* Schoolchildren carry more germs than adults do, partly because of their weaker immune systems, and partly because they come into contact with lots of sick kids. If the children might be coming down with something, leave them home.
- *Be considerate of roommates.* If your loved one's roommate is at risk, do what you can to help (don't visit if you're sick, try to meet in a common area rather than the room). Wouldn't you want others to do the same for your loved one?
- *Avoid crowds during flu season.* Even if you and your loved one are both healthy, you're taking a chance if you head into a crowd (a busy mall, a crowded restaurant) while on an off-grounds trip during flu season.
- *Leave Rover at home.* Few animal-borne diseases are transmitted to humans, but pets, especially dogs, often pick up "human" germs and pass them along to others. Don't bring Rover to the nursing home when an illness is underway.

Dementias and other neurological syndromes

Neurological disorders fall into two general categories: *narrow syndromes* (which target specific parts of the brain and nervous system) and more *widespread syndromes* (which affect multiple brain areas). *Parkinson's disease*—which destroys the brain structures that coordinate fine motor movement—falls into the "narrow" category. In the early stages of Parkinson's disease, the patient develops tremors and balance problems; as the disease progresses, memory and information-processing difficulties begin to emerge. Parkinson's disease is usually treated with medication. (Neural transplants are promising but still years away.) And if your loved one is being treated for Parkinson's disease, be aware. These medications can be difficult to balance precisely and occasionally cause some alarming side effects (such as visual hallucinations). You should alert nursing home staff immediately if any such symptoms occur.

Dementias fall into the other category: They are neurological syndromes with widespread, far-reaching effects. Dementias impair memory, language processing, and a whole host of other cognitive skills. Most dementias take one of three forms:

- *Vascular or multi-infarct dementias* are caused by breakage or blockage of blood vessels that nourish the brain and central nervous system. Because vascular dementias usually follow one or more strokes, high blood pressure and/or cardiac and vascular disorders are significant risk factors.
- *Alzheimer's type dementias*—which result from brain disease

---

DELIRIUM: "TEMPORARY" DEMENTIA

In older adults, certain medications and medical conditions can cause short-term confusion and memory impairment—a condition known as *delirium*. If managed properly, delirium usually clears in a short time. No problem. The problem occurs when delirium is misdiagnosed as dementia, which happens less than it used to, but more than it should. If your loved one seems disoriented and confused, take note. The following signs suggest delirium rather than dementia:

- Confusion and disorientation onset rapidly—in a matter of minutes or hours rather than days or weeks.
- Problems onset after a new medication is introduced, or after a change in medication dosage or timing.
- Problems begin postsurgery or after a medical procedure.
- Symptoms wax and wane in concert with other disease processes.

rather than stroke—are less common than vascular dementias, though they have gotten considerable attention in both
the medical and lay communities in recent years. (We discussed Alzheimer's type dementias in Chapter 2.)
* *Injury-based dementias* result from head injuries (both minor
and major), though the symptoms may not appear for years—
sometimes decades—following the injuries. A series of
concussions early in life increases dementia risk later in life.

Cancers

Cancers result from unusual cell growth and proliferation: The body begins producing mutated cells at a rapid rate, and these fast-growing cancer
cells eventually overwhelm the healthy cells. Any organ system can be affected, and under certain conditions, cancer in one area of the body may
metastasize, releasing cells that flow through the blood and lymph systems to
other areas of the body. Cancers can also set the stage for other diseases by
speeding organ breakdown. (For example, liver cancer can lead to jaundice.)

Risk for many types of cancer increases with age; prostate cancer (in
men), and skin and colorectal cancers (in both women and men) are particularly common among nursing home residents. Cancers are usually treated
by a combination of surgery, chemotherapy, and radiation, but because cell
growth (including cancer cell growth) is slower in older adults, oftentimes
late-life cancers are managed with "watchful waiting" in lieu of more aggressive treatments. In the later stages of the disease, cancer patients often
need extensive pain management, accomplished through medications and
other therapies (such as relaxation).

Joint diseases

Osteoarthritis (thinning of friction-reducing cartilage in the joints) and
rheumatoid arthritis (joint damage caused by the body's own immune system) are common in nursing home residents. So are degenerative joint and
disc disease, gout, and bursitis. It is a rare (and lucky) older adult who does
not suffer from at least one of these painful conditions.

Joint diseases have many different causes, but they all result in impaired
movement—a serious problem for older adults. In fact, impaired movement
stemming from joint disease underlies much of the ADL deterioration that

occurs in nursing homes. (If you can't move, you can't bathe.) Effective pain management is key for the joint disease patient: When pain is reduced, usually through a combination of medication and exercise, movement becomes ███████, ███ ADL █ ███ ███████████

Skin problems

When a person doesn't move much, his or her body weight tends to press on the same areas most of the time. This constant pressure erodes the skin and restricts blood flow to the affected area. Skin cells die, and the skin loses much of its elasticity. *Pressure sores* (also called "bedsores") can develop into ulcers that eat through the skin, sometimes becoming quite deep. (On occasion, an untreated ulcer will reach all the way to the bone.) When ulcers develop, the patient is in a life-threatening situation: Gangrene and other diseases may follow, and once they begin, they're difficult to treat because of the older adult's inefficient immune system. (Something else you need to know about ulcers: They smell unbelievably bad—like rotting flesh—so be prepared for this if your loved one develops a skin ulcer.)

To minimize pressure sores and ulcers, bed- and chair-bound patients must be repositioned frequently, using proper methods. (Aides are trained to do this.) Their skin must kept dry and clean. If an open wound does develop, a vacuum-assisted closure device or "wound vac" may be used to close the wound and speed the healing process. (Wound vacs work by applying negative pressure through a tube embedded in a foam dressing that is sealed to the skin, thereby removing excess liquid and dead tissue.) Nursing staff are usually glad to explain the purposes and procedures of these and other treatments; just ask.

Vascular and cardiac diseases

The body's blood vessels (and there are literally miles of them) are prone to myriad problems, including blockage, breakage, ballooning, and hardening. *Hypertension* (high blood pressure) can lead to stroke (see the earlier section on *dementias*), and it may affect the heart's ability to pump blood to various organs, including itself. When inefficient kidneys allow waste products to build up, the electrical activity of the heart is compromised, and *arrhythmia* (irregular heartbeat) can occur.

Blood clots, congestive heart failure (caused by a decline in blood flow to the heart), bundle branch blockages (blockages of the nerves that regulate heartbeat), and infarcts (heart attacks) are common among nursing home residents. These conditions are treated with various combinations of surgery (to unclog or repair broken vessels), pacemakers (to regulate heart rhythms), medication (to regulate the heartbeat or alter blood pressure), and diet and exercise regimens (to prevent further damage).

Metabolic and endocrine diseases

Adult-onset diabetes is probably the most common *endocrine* (hormonal) disease in nursing home residents: Unable to metabolize blood glucose (blood sugar) effectively, the diabetic patient's body is deprived of nutrients, and cells die in various organ systems (most notably the eyes and circulatory system). Thyroid disease ("Grave's disease") can cause the patient's metabolism to speed up (if the thyroid gland is overactive), or slow down (if the thyroid is underactive). The symptoms of diabetes, thyroid disease, and other metabolic illnesses are usually managed through medication, diet, and exercise, though occasionally more aggressive interventions —like radiation treatment or surgery for thyroid disease—are needed.

Diseases of the eye

Three eye diseases are particularly common in older adults:

- *Cataracts* (clouding of the cornea, the clear film that covers the pupil) underly much of the ADL decline in older adults, and once significant clouding has occurred, surgery may be needed to restore lost vision.
- *Glaucoma* results from loss of blood vessels in the retina—the light-sensitive film at the back of the eyeball. Often a byproduct of diabetes, glaucoma almost always results in at least some vision loss. Left untreated, it can lead to blindness. Glaucoma can be managed by medication, though for many people, the best treatment is prevention. Careful management of illnesses, like diabetes, helps to prevent glaucoma in the first place.

• *Macular degeneration* is caused by leakage in the retina's blood vessels, which leads to an ever-widening blind spot in the center of the visual field. Macular degeneration has traditionally been treated via surgery to replace or repair leaky vessels, but laser and drug treatments have begun to yield promising results.

Pulmonary disease

Chronic obstructive pulmonary disease (COPD) is common among nursing home residents; other lung diseases, like asthma and emphysema, may also occur. All lung diseases produce a similar result: Unable to obtain adequate oxygen, the person is short of breath and energy. They may be completely "winded" by the simplest movement—just sitting upright is a tremendous effort. Fleeting confusion, palpitations (racing heart), and panic are not unusual if the brain becomes oxygen-deprived.

A variety of medications (many delivered by inhaler or nebulizer) are used to enhance oxygen absorption by widening the airways or increasing blood flow to the lungs. Supplemental oxygen may also be delivered via an oxygen tent, or nasal cannula (air tube that sends oxygen into the nostrils). Once lung disease has onset, the lungs sometimes lose the capacity to eliminate byproducts efficiently, leading to *pneumonia*—a buildup of fluid in the lung tissues. Suction may be needed to eliminate the fluids.

Renal and urinary disorders

These fall into three categories:

• *Blockages.* Because the kidneys work less efficiently with age, wastes are not removed as quickly or as completely. When wastes and other byproducts linger in the body, they sometimes form calculi ("stones"), that cause pain and infection, or even block passages entirely. Surgical and microwave procedures are the treatments of choice for calculi and other blockages.

• *Infections.* The aging urinary tract becomes vulnerable to bacterial infection, especially in women. Urinary tract infections can be extremely painful; left untreated, they can be dangerous as well. Urinary tract infections can spread to the kidneys, and if the kidneys begin to fail, dialysis (a mechanical "laundering" process) is needed to filter and clean the blood.

• *Urinary retention and incontinence.* In men, the prostate gland may enlarge to the point that it closes off the urethra (urinary passage); urination becomes difficult—sometimes impossible—and urinary retention results. Women often have the opposite problem: Standing, walking, sneezing, laughing—any and all can cause involuntary urine leakage. Medication, surgery, and catheterization help minimize the symptoms of an enlarged prostate in men; in women, Kegel exercises and adult diapers help manage urinary incontinence.

Digestive/elimination difficulties

As the body processes food less efficiently, a variety of digestive problems can develop. (These are often exacerbated by medications used to treat other, unrelated illnesses.) *Diverticulosis* (outpouchings in the intestinal wall) can lead to discomfort, sometimes infection. When organs that assist in the digestive process no longer work properly (as in gallbladder disease), certain foods become difficult to digest. Diet must be modified to accomodate this; in severe cases, gallbladder surgery may be needed.

When the valves that separate different sections of the digestive tract no longer close completely, corrosive digestive acids can "backwash" onto delicate tissues. *Reflux disease* (leakage of stomach acid into the esophagus) is common. Medication, a change in meal schedules (so the person doesn't eat close to bedtime), and elevating the head of the bed a few inches (to minimize stomach acid backwash at night) can help manage the symptoms of reflux disease.

Peristalsis (muscle movements needed to push digested food along) can become weak and irregular in later life—constipation or bowel blockage ("impaction") are fairly common. Enemas, medication, and diet changes—alone or in combination—are often effective in minimizing constipation and bowel blockage problems. (Some older adults have the opposite problem: When the rectum and anus function less efficiently, fecal incontinence can occur, and adult diapers are needed.)

SOURCES OF INFORMATION ON LATE-LIFE ILLNESS

Here are resources you can use to obtain cutting edge information on late-life medical problems. (We provide additional medical resources—for these and other illnesses—in the Resource and Contact Information section at the back of the book.)

Alzheimer's disease	Alzheimer's Association 225 North Michigan Avenue Chicago, IL 60601 800-272-3900 www.alz.org
Arthritis	Arthritis Foundation P.O. Box 7669 Atlanta, GA 30357 800-283-7800 www.arthritis.org
Cancer	National Cancer Institute Public Inquiries Office 6116 Executive Boulevard, Room 3036A Bethesda, MD 20892 800-4-CANCER www.cancer.gov
Diabetes	American Diabetes Association 1701 North Beauregard Street Alexandria, VA 22311 800-342-2383 www.diabetes.org
Eye disease	American Academy of Ophthalmology P.O. Box 7424 San Francisco, CA 94120 415-561-8500 www.aao.org

Heart disease	American Heart Association 7272 Greenville Avenue Dallas, TX 75231 800-242-8721 www.americanheart.org
Kidney disease	National Kidney Foundation 30 East 33rd Street New York, NY 10016 800-622-9010 www.kidney.org
Lung disease	American Lung Association 61 Broadway, 6th Floor New York, NY 10006 800-LUNG-USA or 212-315-8700 www.lungusa.org
Osteoporosis	National Osteoporosis Foundation 1232 22nd Street, NW Washington, DC 20037 800-231-4222 or 202-223-2226 www.nof.org
Parkinson's disease	American Parkinson's Disease Association 135 Parkinson Avenue Staten Island, NY 10305 800-223-2732 or 718-981-8001 www.apdaparkinson.org
Stroke	National Institute of Neurological Disorders and Stroke NIH Neurological Institute P.O. Box 5801 Bethesda, MD 20824 800-352-9424 www.ninds.nih.gov

OBSTACLES TO
ACCURATE DIAGNOSIS

Most nursing home physicians are experienced at diagnosing medical problems in older adults, but no one can be right 100 percent of the time. Here are some obstacles to accurate diagnosis:

- *Uncooperative patient.* The findings are clear: Patient cooperativeness enhances diagnostic accuracy. When the sullen patient gives cursory, superficial responses, the physician may not have enough information to make a good assessment. The demented patient may be unable to provide any sort of cohesive report at all, so observations made by nursing staff become even more valuable.
- *Inaccurate history.* When the patient provides little information, the physician must rely on family members for accurate data. Here's where you can contribute: Gather whatever information you have about your loved one's medical history, and bring notes along, plus documents (test reports, etc.), if you have them. Ask your loved one's previous physician to forward information to the nursing home physician if a switch was made upon entering the facility.
- *Context.* When a person is in a nursing home, physicians often "expect" to see symptoms of dementia and misinterpret behaviors accordingly (hence, the delirium-dementia problem). Events within the facility can also undermine diagnostic accuracy. (A flu epidemic may cause the physician to ignore alternative diagnoses when a patient exhibits flu-like symptoms.) Always ask the doctor what alternative diagnoses might be considered and why she ruled these out.

Why Treat It If You Can't Make It Better?

Advances in medicine have spoiled us: We're less tolerant than ever of illness and disease—as if everything should be curable, and all treatments painless. Nursing homes are filled with residents and family members who insist that physicians and staff "fix" the unfixable, and then assume that all treatment failures are due to the doctor's incompetence or the staff's negligence.

MEDICAL INFORMATION ON THE INTERNET: A WORD OF WARNING

It's difficult to distinguish accurate from inaccurate information on the Internet—especially where health-related topics are concerned. When researching late-life health issues online, stick to web sites created by reputable organizations like the American Medical Association or National Institutes of Health, and avoid those associated with private, for-profit companies. Warning signs of a poorly run or dishonest web site include:

- promises of a "miracle" or "can't fail" treatment
- a great deal of space devoted to advertising particular products or services (usually the company's)
- requests for personal information for follow-up mailings or telephone solicitations
- infrequent updating with new information (the date of a web site's most recent revision is usually listed at the bottom of the opening page)
- a slanted, biased perspective (often indicated by attacks on competitors or traditional treatment approaches)

In part, these attitudes stem from our unwillingness to accept the inevitability of illness and death—in ourselves, or in someone we love. (We'll take up this issue in Chapter 12.) Your challenge, as a caregiver, is to be kind but realistic: You and your loved one must decide when aggressive—sometimes painful—interventions are warranted, and when it's best to take a less aggressive approach. Here are some key issues to consider:

- *Maintenance versus cure.* "Quality of life" is an elusive concept—hard to define, even harder to measure. Sometimes a treatment can be worse than the illness itself, and in such situations it may be better to maintain the status quo than go all out to "fix" the problem. If the choice comes down to painful treatment versus death, most, but not all, people opt for treatment—at least at the outset. More common is the situation where a disease process can't be reversed, but physicians can manage the symptoms and keep the person reasonably comfortable. Remember: In long term care, maximizing comfort and independence are legitimate treatment goals. Helping your loved one focus on how well he's held the line, instead of fretting about his failure to improve, is the best thing you can do in many situations.

• *Accepting and accommodating what we can't change.* Most people are surprisingly adaptive: They find ways to get by, if given a chance. People survive—even thrive—despite lost limbs, failing eyesight and hearing, an inability to eat or speak...you name it. When losses mount, the patient's greatest hurdle may be accepting the reality of the situation and learning to work with what's available. Acceptance takes time and cannot be rushed, but focusing on the past won't do anyone any good. If you must cry when you think about Dad's amputated foot, do it on your own time. When you're with him, be strong. Your job is to motivate him—to help him make it back to his seat at the stadium once he's gotten the hang of his new prosthesis. But he'll only make it if you support and encourage him.

• *Appropriate treatment makes problems more manageable.* Many folks believe that once disease hits, it's over. They might as well do as they wish (so they say)—Why bother with the hassles of treatment? Family members sometimes reinforce this way of thinking, sneaking cigarettes to the emphysema patient or sweets to the diabetic. (They rationalize this by arguing that they "can't take away [the patient's] only pleasure.") Don't conspire with your loved one to undermine his fragile health. Your well-meaning actions can only lead to further complications and a worsening situation. You might not be able to cure your mother's diabetes, but you can help her manage the symptoms and avoid the more serious consequences of the disease, like blindness and limb loss.

• *Small improvements make big differences.* When family members first hear about the modest goals set by nursing home treatment teams, they sometimes assume that the staff are

WHAT'S *THAT* FOR?
MEDICAL EQUIPMENT IN THE NURSING HOME

If you've spent much time in hospitals, you know that one of the most unsettling aspects of treatment is the equipment: monitors, tubes, syringes, and bags—sometimes so numerous they make it hard to see the patient. Here's some of what you'll encounter when you visit the nursing home:

- *Catheters* are tubes that drain fluid from the body. They are often used in patients with bladder problems. Properly inserted, catheters don't hurt, but they can be difficult to maneuver and a bit frightening-looking as well.
- *Feeding tubes* are inserted into the patient's stomach through a small surgically-developed opening in the abdomen. They allow liquid nutrients to be fed directly into the stomach, and temporary feeding tubes are common in patients who are learning to eat again after a stroke.
- *Fistulas* (also called "ports") are surgically made entry points used to connect blood vessels with frequently used medical equipment (such as dialysis machines). Fistulas are usually permanent, and once healed, they don't hurt, but like catheters, they take some getting used to.
- *Gerichairs* (or "posture chairs") are reclining chairs on wheels, used to transport folks who can't sit in a wheelchair because of postural problems or agitation. Gerichairs are comfortable (like a regular recliner), but difficult to exit without assistance. This is intentional: They're made so the patient doesn't fall out of them.
- *Nasal cannulas* are tubes leading from oxygen tanks to the patient's nose. Unlike oxygen masks, they allow the person to eat and speak freely (though some patients complain of feeling constrained by them, particularly if they are not used to wearing glasses or having anything on or near their face).
- *Tracheotomy tubes* are inserted through a surgically developed hole in the patient's throat to facilitate breathing. The tube doesn't hurt, but it may become uncomfortable when clogged (which happens fairly often).
- *Trapezes* are pulleys and handles suspended over the patient's bed or chair. They are designed to help those with muscle weakness or partial paralysis shift positions by themselves, and they're harder to use than they look.

either nitpicky or crazy (or both). These people are going to spend weeks teaching a ninety-year-old cancer patient to use a walker? If this seems like a waste of time, remember: small gains can make a tremendous difference in a person's quality of life. To the bed- or wheelchair-bound resident, the prospect of using a walker to get to the bathroom on their own sounds wonderful. It might take a lot of effort to achieve small gains, but small gains are important to the person who's making them. Little things really do mean a lot where illnesses and disabilities are concerned.

10

A Realistic Approach to Behavior Problems: No More Peeing in the Petunias

2/14/08: Nursing Notes, Mr. Ronald Everhardt.

7:12 A.M. Pt AWOL from morning meal—interior and exterior search initiated. Pt found on bench in sitting area near parking lot B, confused but responsive, wearing pjs + bathrobe. Stated upon questioning that he was "waiting for breakfast." Pt dressed in room (w/assistance), then led to dining hall. Compliant, mood generally positive; meal uneventful.

8:55 A.M. Pt discovered in Rm. 1-12 (custodial closet), partially disrobed. Led easily to common area; soc services (L. Durbin) calmed + reoriented pt. (see soc svc doc.)

9:50 A.M. Pt at nurses' station, w/vague complains of "pain" "hurts" "can't go." Upon quest., pt reported burning/itching sensation when urinating. Consult ASAP to r/o urinary tract infection, STD. Dietary consult 2/14 P.M. or 2/15 A.M., per Dr. Mendelsohn.

11:30 A.M. Pt at nurses' station, moderate agitation. Complains of burning, increased pain at urination. Urology consult scheduled 4 P.M. today, post OT, dietary.

2:45 P.M. Pt refusing OT, increased agitation, reports of intense pain/burning. Paged Dr. Mendelsohn; lft msg.

3:40 P.M. Pt AWOL from scheduled dietary consult; found upon exterior search, urinating in flowerbed near entrance sitting (bench) area. Combative upon approach. Pt returned to common area after ~5 min; calm w/aides, less confused. Soiled clothing, bedclothes changed.

4:40 P.M. Urology consult to r/o UTI, STD. Probable UTI. Eryth 400 mg TID initial; reassess 72 hr. No other med changes. Continue OT, PT. (see consult urol note)

9:50 P.M. Evening meal, post-meal interactions uneventful. Pt generally compliant; mood mixed, continued complaints re itching/burning (intermittent). Calmed by TV, common area activities. In bed at ~9:00.

When nursing home residents develop behavior problems, the entire facility suffers. Behavior problems drain staff members' time, sap their energy, and hasten turnover and burnout. Behavior problems stress the residents, worsen their symptoms, and decrease their quality of life. Last but not least, behavior problems can alienate family members, young and old alike. Visits become less pleasant and less frequent.

In this chapter, we discuss common behavior problems in nursing home residents. We describe how behavior problems are addressed by nursing home staff, what you should do if your loved one exhibits any of these problems, and how you can maintain a good relationship with your loved one in the face of his or her challenging behavior.

Behavior Problems: Causes and Treatments

Behavior problems in nursing homes usually result from four factors, alone or in combination. These are:

- *Cognitive decline.* Dementia and stroke impair judgment and memory; confusion and disinhibition (with their associated behavioral difficulties) usually follow.
- *Environmental factors.* Too much (or too little) stimulation, troublesome neighbors, staffing problems—these and other environmental factors can lead to behavior problems in an otherwise placid resident.
- *Inadequately treated pain or illness.* Inadequately treated pain or illness causes fatigue and irritability; unless the underlying problem is addressed, behavioral difficulties usually ensue.
- *Psychological factors.* Depression and anxiety (both common in nursing home residents) contribute to a whole host of behavior problems—from wandering and aggressiveness to withdrawal and self-destructive, even suicidal behavior.

Like causes, most treatments for behavior problems fall into four categories:

- *Behavioral interventions.* Though the specifics differ from situation to situation, the basics of behavioral treatments (also called *behavior modification techniques*) are always the same: A problem behavior is identified, the factors that reinforce (encourage) that behavior are found, and interventions are used to remove those reinforcing factors.
- *Environmental changes.* When the environment is the problem, environmental changes can make a world of difference. If an Alzheimer's patient becomes confused and agitated by the sound of multiple TV sets, relocating that person to a quiet area can go a long way toward solving the problem.

- *Medication.* Medication helps eliminate problem behavior by alleviating its underlying cause—whether the cause is psychological (like depression) or physical (like a bladder infection).
- *Psychological interventions.* Older adults are often quite receptive to psychotherapy, though they may be guarded and suspicious at the outset. In combination with medication, psychotherapy can be an effective treatment for depression, anxiety, and other emotional difficulties.

CAN MEDICATION REALLY SLOW THE PROGRESS OF ALZHEIMER'S DISEASE?

You've probably seen the advertisements on TV: new medications that help counter the confusion and memory loss associated with Alzheimer's disease. These medications (called *cholinesterase inhibitors)* all work the same way, by increasing the brain's supply of acetylcholine, a neurotransmitter critical for good cognitive function. Taken during the early stages of Alzheimer's disease, cholinesterase inhibitors may actually improve memory and other cognitive functions (such as language use). In the middle and later stages of the disease, cholinesterase inhibitors don't improve functioning, but stabilize and slow the rate of decline. Side effects of cholinesterase inhibitors are generally fairly mild (stomach upset, insomnia).

Keep in mind that the effectiveness of these medications tends to fade after two to three years—so they don't solve the problem of Alzheimer's disease, but may temporarily slow its progression. More long-term studies are needed before the benefits and limitations of cholinesterase inhibitors are fully understood.

Common Behavior Problems in Nursing Home Residents

Every person is different, but certain behavior problems emerge again and again in nursing homes. You might not see these in your loved one, but chances are you'll see some of them in other nursing home residents.

Insulting and accusing others

When illness-related discomfort meets up with dementia-based disinhibition, fireworks often ensue. People in pain tend to lash out at others, and on occasion some pretty nasty insults make their way into a resident's angry commentary—an unpleasant, awkward situation for everyone. Awkward situations also arise when a demented resident blames every misplaced sock on the thievery of roommates or nursing staff. (This happens more than you might think.)

When insults and accusations are truly a byproduct of dementia, the best response is to ignore them. (Easier said than done when the target is you.) In these situations, staff will counsel other residents to try to let the insults and accusations go unchallenged—to "walk away" rather than argue or rebut.

It's different when the behavior is under the resident's control. In this situation, staff usually begin by advising the person that others find her remarks hurtful and unacceptable, and that there may be consequences if the behavior continues. Sometimes the problem is due to ignorance: The individual really doesn't know how to behave around others. (This is most common in people who have lived an isolated existence for many years.) Effective interventions include modeling the proper behavior (staff may do this) or directing the resident's attention to a more socially skilled peer.

Wandering

Many demented residents cope with restlessness by walking. Confusion and memory problems prevent them from finding their way back to where they started, and rather than asking directions (which might not make sense to them anyway), they just keep on moving, hoping that a familiar face or landmark will emerge to put everything into perspective.

MEMORY BOXES

Some nursing homes use *memory boxes* (also called *locator boxes*) to help reorient confused residents. A memory box is an eye-level display case with clear front and sides, placed directly outside the resident's room. It is filled with personal possessions (old photos, ID cards, work-related objects), and serves as a kind of landmark for residents—a sign that they've found their way "home" again. When memory boxes are used, wandering, stealing, and other behavioral problems decrease. If your loved one's nursing home doesn't use memory boxes, suggest that they start.

If your loved one is wandering, she probably needs to be in a secure setting. Many homes have bracelet alarm systems to alert staff when a resident is going AWOL, but this is an imperfect solution: Busy staff might not be able to stop what they're doing to intercept a confused resident heading toward a busy highway.

Happily, today's secure settings bear little resemblance to the "locked units" of the past. In newer facilities, residents may have access to miles of walkways and paths, both indoors and out, though the exit points are carefully monitored. Many facilities also use color-codes and other easy-to-identify cues to reorient confused residents. Some nursing homes help residents burn excess energy on treadmills and stationary bikes, or in exercise classes tailored to their physical limitations.

Stealing

Things get stolen in nursing homes, but "theft" by residents is usually a byproduct of dementia-based confusion: The person sees something that looks vaguely familiar, assumes it's his, and takes it. It's easy to misinterpret this as theft, but most of the time, the confused resident simply picks up an item, wanders off with it, realizes it isn't his, and leaves it somewhere.

Anything and everything can get "stolen" in this way. (Nursing home staff usually have a story or two about missing false teeth that magically appeared on the wrong nightstand—or in the wrong mouth!) There's no way to eliminate stealing completely in a setting where privacy is at a premium.

SLEEP DISRUPTION AND BEHAVIORAL DIFFICULTIES

Sleep problems are common in nursing home residents, and can set the stage for wandering and aggressiveness. In many instances, sleep problems stem from medication side effects, but sometimes sleep problems signal underlying depression or anxiety. Insomnia can also result from situational factors—being in an unfamiliar place without the usual bedtime and morning cues (the sound of the heater going on, a spouse's familiar snore).

When sleep patterns are disrupted, medical and psychological factors must first be ruled out. If problems persist, daytime activity levels should be increased, so the person is tired by evening. A "sleep hygiene" program can be set up to eliminate insomnia-producing behaviors (like drinking coffee with dinner). If all else fails, staff may have to work with the resident during sleepless periods, to keep him occupied and monitored.

The best you can do is label things clearly, and keep valuable objects locked and secure. Tolerance and a bit of good humor help, too.

Hoarding

Hoarding is common in nursing homes, particularly among residents raised in households that lacked the basics. Sometimes a resident will hoard something in her room (most often food or paper supplies), so she doesn't "run out." If these materials are neatly organized, it's not so bad. But when they're jammed into every drawer and stuffed beneath the mattress, these stockpiles can become dangerous. (Paper becomes a fire hazard; food attracts vermin.) The problem can usually be addressed by allowing the resident to keep a private stock of whatever she's worried about, for her use only—if she'll promise to keep it tidy and organized.

Aggression

When a confused person feels threatened or intruded upon, instinct takes over, and he may strike out to defend himself. To make matters worse, residents are often "armed"—with canes, walkers, or other assistive devices that double as weapons. Make no mistake: Residents can—and do—direct physical aggression toward staff, other residents, and visitors.

The key to managing aggression lies in identifying its causes or "triggers." When staff analyze the situation closely, they'll usually discover a pattern—particular events that tend to occur right before the outbursts. The best way to deal with aggression is to prevent it before it occurs: Identify a resident's triggers and keep them from occurring in his presence.

Repetitive questioning and repetitious behavior

Some dementia patients exhibit *behavioral stereotypy*—they repeat the same question, statement, or behavior (like pacing), over and over again, for hours, days, or weeks on end. They're not doing this deliberately: In most cases, they genuinely cannot stop the behavior. Behavioral stereotypy is thought to stem from deterioration of those parts of the brain that provide a feeling of closure after having completed an action or gotten the answer to a question. It is truly beyond the person's control.

As you might guess, the experience is often distressing to the patient, who feels anxious and "stuck," and can sometimes become quite agitated. The experience is also distressing for those nearby, who may find themselves harangued with the same question hundreds of times in the course of an hour. This can be vexing when the question is delivered calmly, but when it's being shouted by someone in an agitated state, it's nearly unbearable.

Not surprisingly, repetitive questioning often triggers aggression in other residents, who become frustrated when the person won't leave them alone. For this reason, the behavior usually elicits a rapid response from nursing home staff, who initiate medical and psychiatric consultations, along with behavioral and environmental interventions to stop the behavior.

What should you do if you become the focus of your loved one's repetitive questioning? First, respond to the question once or twice. If your answer clearly isn't penetrating, see if you can distract her by changing the subject or beginning a new activity (like taking a walk). And don't be upset with yourself if you feel completely frazzled after a barrage of repetitive questions—even seasoned nursing home veterans report feeling this way.

Refusing to eat

Despite the Dietary Staff's best efforts (favorite foods, extra goodies, special eating arrangements), sometimes a nursing home resident simply refuses to eat or drink. Refusing to drink is the more serious of the two. While many people can go without eating for a while, refusal to take in fluids can lead to serious health problems in a very short time.

When a resident refuses to eat or drink, staff will notify the resident's physician who'll assess the situation and look for a physical cause, such as infection or a bowel obstruction. If no physical basis for the behavior can be found, a psychiatric consultation usually follows. Appetite loss and refusal to drink are common symptoms of depression in older adults. If depression is the cause, the psychiatrist may recommend antidepressant medication and possibly psychotherapy as well.

Noncompliance

As we discussed in Chapter 8, nursing home residents have the right to refuse treatments or decline to take part in most activities. They also have the right to discontinue a treatment or activity, even after they've started it. However, nursing home residents do *not* have the right to agree to take part in a treatment or activity, and then proceed to fight it off, disrupt it, or sabotage it repeatedly. This behavior (called *noncompliance*) can result in discharge from a service (with all the associated funding headaches) or even discharge from the facility itself if the behavior is interfering with other residents' well-being.

If the noncompliant resident is alert and oriented, the best response is a frank discussion of reasons underlying the behavior. Does he think he'll be able to live with a favorite relative if he gets "kicked out" of the facility? Is this his way of getting attention or asserting himself? Is he refusing because he can't remember what to do and doesn't want to admit this publicly? Sometimes when the underlying reasons are addressed, noncompliant behavior dissipates by itself.

Inappropriate elimination

A mildly demented resident may be oriented enough to know when she needs to use the bathroom, but not remember where the bathroom is (and she may be ashamed to ask). To the more profoundly disoriented resident (like Mr. Everhardt, whose problems we discussed at the start of this chapter), any closed space, like a closet, may be sufficiently "bathroom-like" that it seems a viable option. Because this problem is common in nursing homes,

MOM'S DOING *WHAT* WITH *WHOM*?

To the surprise of many families, nursing homes can be very romantic places. After all, they're filled with lonely people in need of acceptance and affection. Romances are common, and so are purely physical dalliances. Families tend to avoid thinking about residents' sexual needs, but such needs do exist, and they won't go away because you pretend they're not there.

Most of the time, nursing home romances work out fine. The problems arise when one or both participants are unable to give true legal consent to the activity. In this situation, actions do *not* speak louder than words: The fact that a resident is participating (even quite enthusiastically) does not mean they realize exactly what they're doing, or who they're doing it with.

The family's usual response is "Make it stop!", but when the resident's rights to privacy and free association clash with questions of consent, staff feel trapped between a rock and a hard place. If the residents seem happy, staff rarely intervene.

staff usually have a number of interventions in place to deal with it, such as instituting regular toileting intervals and learning the resident's signals so they can steer her toward a bathroom when the time comes.

If inappropriate elimination is not due to dementia, it's usually a result of infection or illness (so staff will check for a urinary tract infection soon after accidents begin). Some illnesses can impair sphincter control as well (as anyone who's had diarrhea knows), and sometimes there's little warning before an accident occurs.

Inappropriate sexual behavior

Again, this is usually a byproduct of dementia—the resident knows what she wants to do but is confused about where, when, and with whom sexual behavior is appropriate. Disrobing and masturbating in public are common in disoriented nursing home residents; sexual assaults against other residents or staff are much less common, but not unheard of.

When public disrobing or masturbation are taking place, the difficulties have mostly to do with others' reactions (fear, embarrassment, etc.). The resident herself may be stunningly unperturbed. Redirection to a private room and refocusing on a different activity are the interventions of choice in such situations. You can't stop the behavior, but you can channel it to an appropriate location.

Hidden Factors That Set the Stage for Problems

Behavior problems sometimes result from subtle, "hidden" factors—aspects of the environment, or even the treatment, that inadvertently make things worse. These "hidden" factors include:

Inadequate staffing

In a perfect world, nursing home staff would be able to give their undivided attention to each resident, monitoring her triggers, engaging her in constructive activities, and soothing her as needed. In the real world, there simply aren't enough staff on hand to do this. In many facilities, staff attention is taken up more-or-less completely with basic resident care, and there's little time left for dealing with behavioral problems.

Sensory overload

As we age, we lose the ability to screen out irrelevant information, especially when we're bombarded by sights and sounds from multiple sources. Stroke and dementia further impair our "information screening" abilities, which can make a nursing home a pretty overwhelming place. Ironically, the very factors that make a nursing home safe for someone with decreased perceptual acuity—bright lights, loud voices, amplified sounds—can make it hellish for someone who's easily overloaded. The result: Confusion, agitation, and increased aggressiveness. (The good news is that sensory stimulation can be decreased with proper planning, and residents likely to become upset in peak traffic areas can be scheduled for quiet activity in calmer settings.)

Boredom

Nature really does abhor a vacuum. Folks with too much time on their hands tend to develop behavioral problems as a way of getting stimulation in a too-quiet world. This is especially common in alert and oriented residents who lack physical mobility. Quite literally "stuck," they direct their energies toward whatever's nearby (including an easily-agitated peer). Good programming can do a lot to address this problem: A busy resident is rarely bored.

Medication problems

Medication-related behavior problems are surprisingly common. Oftentimes the correct medication is being used but at the wrong dosage. Psychoactive medications, like antidepressants, are particularly difficult to titrate on ill or elderly residents—too little does nothing, too much can be sedating. Sometimes medications interact to cause confusion or aggression, even if neither drug alone would produce this effect. Nursing home staff are usually good at identifying medication-based behavior problems, and they'll act quickly, in concert with the attending physician, to address the issue.

The wrong neighbors

Bad neighbors are a nightmare for anyone, but especially for the nursing home resident. Imagine having a demented neighbor who screams all night, a confused roommate who climbs into bed with you repeatedly, or a wandering peer who walks away with your cherished photo or costly hearing aid. When you complain, you're told the offender "can't help it," or "doesn't know any better." The final insult: You're asked to be patient and understanding, while all the attention goes to the culprit!

Saints have cracked under less pressure. Exposed to the wrong neighbors, even the calmest, most stable people become depressed and anxious, and sometimes verbally or physically aggressive as well.

Knowing When to Call In the Experts

Some behavior problems are best managed over time, and if it takes a few days or weeks to get things under control, that's OK. Other behavior problems require a quick response. Here's how to tell the difference:

Signs that a quick response is needed

Everybody has the occasional bad day, but some behaviors should trigger an immediate reaction by staff. These include:

- refusing to eat or drink
- becoming physically aggressive
- suddenly becoming confused, agitated, or disoriented
- any sudden, severe mood change (usually depression, but a sudden "up" or irritable mood can be worrisome as well)

If your loved one shows any of these signs, staff should (and usually will) take immediate action, alerting the physician, and you as well. You'll need to take a more active role in alerting staff to the subtler changes in your loved one's behavior—things they might not be able to detect until they know her well. Let staff know if your loved one shows any of the following signs:

- withdraw from usual activities
- changes in interpersonal interaction patterns
- increased jumpiness or irritability
- increased worry about unlikely or unrealistic things
- frequent references to their own death

What you should do

Begin by talking with your loved one (unless they are too confused to do this). When you're done, you can share your insights with staff. The nature of the problem will determine who you should go to, but when in doubt, approach the charge nurse. State the problem clearly and calmly, voice your proposed solutions if you have any, and ask what can be done. If

SYMPTOMS OF DEPRESSION
IN OLDER ADULTS

Depression is common in people of all ages, but especially so in older adults. Here are the major symptoms:

- sadness or tearfulness
- feelings of helplessness and hopelessness
- loss of interest and pleasure in usual pursuits
- withdrawal from social contact
- insomnia and easy fatigue
- decreased appetite and weight loss
- impaired concentration and difficulty making decisions
- exaggerated guilt about past mistakes and personal flaws
- preoccupation with death

the problem is serious, a care plan meeting may be called. Be there so you can take an active role in addressing the problem.

What staff will do

After meeting with the patient, the physician may begin a trial of medication, or she may refer the patient to a mental health professional for consultation. If this happens, the patient will likely be interviewed by a psychologist, who will also review the patient's medical records, speak with staff, and observe the patient to identify possible triggers for the problem behaviors. The psychologist will make suggestions about the types of therapy that might help with the problem and may recommend environmental changes to minimize triggers. Sometimes the psychologist will call in a psychiatrist, who may make further suggestions about medications and other treatments.

Families are often surprised that the psychiatrist isn't called in right away, particularly when medication seems the obvious solution. Most of the time, this delay isn't the physician's fault—it's a response to state and federal laws regarding "least restrictive treatments" (which we discussed in Chapter 8). Because psychoactive medication is considered a "chemical restraint," it can be used only when less restrictive interventions have failed unless there are clear risks in delaying treatment. If a psychologist assesses the patient and agrees that a medication consult is warranted, the facility will proceed quickly. However, staff cannot move directly to this more restrictive level of care without a clear recommendation. If they do, they'll face some pretty sharp questions during the next state review.

The Suicidal Nursing Home Patient

Suicide risk increases with age, and older white males are at greatest risk. Nursing home staff are alert to signs of suicidal behavior in residents, but you should be aware of these as well. Here's what to look for, and what to do:

What to look for

Many of the same symptoms that would be worrisome in a younger person emerge in suicidal older adults:

- loss of interest in usual activities and relationships
- diminished sense of hopefulness
- feeling "trapped"—having few options and no good choices
- loss of "future orientation" (no longer talking about the future)
- feeling like a burden to others or that others would be "better off without them"
- talk of suicide (especially when details—like *where*, *when*, and *how* plans—are mentioned)
- *any* type of self-harmful behavior (no matter how "minor")

What to do

If your loved one is showing signs of suicidal thinking or planning, tell the charge nurse, and ask that she inform the attending physician. The physician will probably institute *suicide precautions* and ask for an urgent psychological or psychiatric evaluation. Suicide precautions involve removing potentially lethal materials (particularly those mentioned by the patient as part of their plan), and checking the patient at fifteen-minute intervals.

If suicide precautions seem inadequate, full *suicide watch* may be instituted—the patient must remain within sight and arm's reach of staff at all times. If the patient needs that level of intense supervision to ensure their

---

PSEUDODEMENTIA

Sometimes depressed people show unusual patterns of symptoms, or what is called a "masked depression." In older adults, masked depression may take the form of *pseudodementia* (literally, "false dementia"). The person looks demented but is in fact depressed. Formal neurological assessment by a psychologist is often needed to distinguish actual dementia from pseudodementia so the proper interventions can be used. Talk with the attending physician if your loved one shows two or more of the following signs:

- Rapid onset of symptoms (true dementia symptoms onset gradually)
- Symptoms remain constant throughout the day (true dementia patients tend to get worse in the evening)
- Specific, detailed complaints (true dementia patients offer mostly vague complaints)
- Symptoms lessen in response to antidepressant medications (true dementia does not respond well to antidepressants)
- Frequent expressions of guilt about their symptoms (common in pseudodementia, but not in true dementia)

safety, the process for admission to a psychiatric service is usually initiated, regardless of whether patient and family agree.

Where suicide is concerned, proper treatment can mean the difference between life and death. Medications and psychotherapy can help a depressed patient see that she has options and hope—choices beyond death for dealing with her problems. When drugs and psychotherapy fail, electroconvulsive therapy (ECT) is sometimes used to treat the most severe forms of depression. (See page 188 for details.)

Maintaining a Good Relationship with the Troubled Loved One

It can be difficult to maintain a positive relationship when your loved one has behavior problems. We tend to see problem behavior as something the person can control (even when we know they can't), and we get annoyed, angry, disgusted...you name it. Here are some tips for maintaining a good relationship with your troubled loved one.

Tips for adult children

- *Don't ignore your feelings.* Behavior problems are frustrating for everyone—the resident, other residents, the staff, and you (especially when the behavior brings late-night phone calls from the charge nurse). Don't pretend this isn't provoking certain feelings—resentment, anger, sadness, and so forth. You mustn't burden your loved one with these feelings, but you'll feel better if you share them with someone—a friend, therapist, or pastor, perhaps.
- *Use your common experiences to create empathy.* If you get angry at your parent who's wandering, screaming, or having bathroom accidents, just remember: Once upon a time, you did these very same things. They stuck by you—now you stick by them.
- *Share the burden.* It's a good time to review the caregiving guidelines we discussed in Chapter 1. If you can share the

ECT: JUST THE FACTS

Electroconvulsive therapy (ECT) is one of the most misunderstood treatment techniques in all of medicine. Here's what we know:

Who is ECT best for?

ECT is a "last ditch" treatment approach—it's used when all other treatments have failed. The ideal candidate for ECT is someone with a severe depression that has not responded to other interventions (like antidepressants and psychotherapy). In such cases, ECT can sometimes produce remarkable results: A patient who had been severely depressed for weeks or months may show tremendous improvement in a very short time.

What's involved?

ECT involves passing a brief burst of electricity through the brain, which causes neurons (brain cells) to fire and release large quantities of neurotransmitters (chemicals that relay information from neuron to neuron). Because the brain's neurons fire in greater numbers than usual during ECT, the patient often experiences a brief seizure. (They don't feel it, though—before the procedure begins they are given general anesthesia, along with a muscle relaxant to minimize the intensity of the seizure.)

How does it work?

No one knows for sure. Some researchers think the therapeutic effects of ECT stem from the release of neurotransmitters during the ECT session; other researchers think the electrical stimulation produces long-term increases in brain-cell activity.

Are there side effects?

This is the most controversial aspect of ECT. Most patients report memory loss for events that took place during the hours just before treatment, but some patients have reported more severe memory problems (memory loss for events that occurred years—even decades—before the procedure). We do know that the side effects are less severe when *unilateral ECT* (where electricity is passed through only one hemisphere) is used in lieu of *bilateral ECT* (where electricity is passed through both brain hemispheres at once).

Where do I get information?

The American Psychiatric Association provides written and online information on ECT (if you access their web site, use the *Search* option, and enter the term *ECT*). They can be reached at:

American Psychiatric Association
1000 Wilson Boulevard, Suite 1825
Arlington, VA 22209
703-907-7300
www.psych.org

caregiving burden with siblings, spouse, or other family members, do it. Your parent's behavior problems will be easier to take when the burden is spread around a bit.

Tips for spouses

- *Get some of your needs met elsewhere.* We can't tell you what to do, but we can gently remind you: You have needs, too, and they haven't gone away. You might not choose to seek physical intimacy with another (though some spouses do), but don't ignore your needs for emotional intimacy. Consider joining a support group so you can talk this out.
- *Don't blame the victim.* If your spouse has dementia, remember: He might not know what he's doing much of the time. If you learn that he's climbed into bed with another resident, made a "pass" at an aide, or exposed himself in public, don't blame him. It's not his fault.
- *Don't take responsibility for your loved one's behavior.* You shouldn't blame a demented loved one for behavior problems, but neither should you take responsibility for these difficulties. Your spouse is in a nursing home because he needs to be—he can't manage on his own. There's no need to feel bad or apologize to the nurses about your spouse's ag-

gressiveness or incontinence. Nursing home staff expect this—it's part of the deal.

Tips for siblings

- *Beware of old, familiar patterns.* Siblings have long histories (longer even than spouses), and old habits die hard. Take a close look at your reactions to you sibling's behavior problems, including how you interact with staff around these issues. Ask yourself: Are old, familiar patterns (rivalry, jealousy) repeating themselves again?
- *Don't take it personally.* Family members in general—and siblings in particular—tend to take behavior problems personally. True, late-night phone calls and weekend emergencies can leave you tearing your hair out, but remember: In a person who's demented or severely depressed, these behaviors are hard to control, and they're not really directed at you (even though it might feel that way).

THE TREATMENT STALEMATE

Conflicts arise when a legally competent resident refuses to comply with treatment. Even when the power of attorney, family, physician, and staff all agree on a particular course of action, there are times when the resident simply won't get on board.

If the patient's well-being requires that she receive a treatment, the physician may take action to override this resistance. When all attempts at gentle (and not-so-gentle) persuasion have failed, the physician can order that the patient be restrained—either chemically or physically—so treatment can proceed. Given the legal implications of involuntary treatment, this is used only as a last resort—but it *will* be used if all else fails.

11

When Things Get Better:
The Transition Back Home

The meeting was about to begin. All around the table, people were chatting and shuffling papers. Barb Callahan walked in, laden with folders and files. One thing you could count on at Harter Hall: The finance people were always the last to arrive. Barb closed the door and took a seat at the far end of the table.

Anne turned to Helen and winked. "You must be excited," she said softly. "You've been looking forward to this for a while."

Helen couldn't help but smile. "Oh, yes," she said, nodding. "I certainly have."

Anne cleared her throat and the room grew quiet. She began.

"OK, let's get started. Helen's been with us since mid-October—eighteen weeks now. She's made outstanding progress, and Dr. Small has asked us to finish discharge planning. Dave?" Dave was Harter Hall's Social Services director.

"Helen will be going to assisted living upon discharge—to Michael Manor. Dr. Small wants follow-ups in place for ongoing diabetes management and an ophthalmology consult."

"Right," said Anne, "the cataracts. Nothing else?"

No one spoke.

Anne looked down at the chart. "Funding?" she said to no one in particular. She scribbled a note on the front of the folder.

"Paperwork's been filed. We've got preliminary approval all around." Barb thumbed through the pages on her clipboard. "I'm waiting on a fax from one of the secondaries," she continued, "but we're ready to go."

Anne put down her pen. She leaned back in her chair. The room was silent. Everyone was waiting for Anne's next question. Instead, she leaned toward Helen, patted her on the arm.

"Well, Helen, this is it. We're certainly going to miss you."

Helen smiled but said nothing. She looked down at the table.

"Why, Helen," said Jill. "I believe you're blushing!"

Helen shook her head slowly. After a moment she looked up, and over at Jill. Her eyes were moist. "Well," she said softly, "I never thought I'd say this, but I'll miss you guys, too."

Everyone was quiet. Someone coughed. After a few moments, Anne broke the silence.

"Helen, you know you can visit us anytime."

Helen nodded.

Anne looked over at the Social Services director. "Dave, when's the date?"

"We're set for Monday—Monday at nine."

Anne closed the chart, placed it on the table. "Monday it is. And we're done."

To the nursing home resident and her family, discharge planning can be the best of times—a formal declaration from nursing home staff that the resident can make it on her own again. But discharge planning can be the worst of times as well, when conflicts arise regarding post–nursing home placement (also called *aftercare*). On occasion, the resident and her family have very different views regarding where she should live and who should provide personal and financial support. These are the challenges of nursing home discharge.

Discharge Settings

Where do people go when they leave a nursing home? Usually to one of four places:

- *Home.* Some residents move back to the same house or apartment they lived in before they entered the nursing home. These are the highest-functioning residents—the ones who have made the most complete recovery. In-home care is often used to facilitate independent living after discharge, especially during the first few weeks. (If this applies to your loved one, you might want to review the home care material in Chapter 3 before discharge planning begins in earnest.)

- *A family member's home.* Some residents move into a family member's home, rather than living alone. These are the residents who have made a good recovery but still need a fair amount of help and support. Some residents move in with family members as a way of making the transition back to their own house or apartment; others stay with family for an extended period (sometimes permanently, or until a higher level of care is needed again).

- *Assisted living.* Some residents never recover enough to resume independent living, even with the family's help. These residents typically move to assisted living following their nursing home stay. As you may remember from Chapter 5, assisted living facilities are designed for people who need help with complex ADLs (bathing, dressing, etc.) and basic medical needs (such as blood sugar monitoring) on a daily basis.

- *Long-term care.* Some residents develop further problems or complications, or are simply unable to regain a degree of independent functioning that would enable them to live at lower levels of care.

Discharge Planning Meetings

When your loved one's independent living skills improve to the point that nursing home care is no longer needed, one or more discharge planning meetings will be scheduled. Important decisions are made at these meetings—decisions that will affect you as well as your loved one. You should attend the first meeting for sure and as many follow-up meetings as you can. As you'll discover, information from three sources—staff, family, and the resident herself—will be used to assess readiness for discharge.

Staff input

In discharge planning meetings, staff members from each department in the nursing home are asked two things:

DISCHARGE PLANNING:
KEY INFORMATION FOR FAMILY MEMBERS

To help your loved one make sound decisions regarding discharge plans, you should gather information regarding your loved one's *functional capacity* and *financial/insurance status*. The information is there for the taking—you just have to ask.

- *Functional capacity.* As discharge approaches, a review of the current care plan will give you a good picture of your loved one's functional capacity. Beyond the care plan itself, a great deal of paperwork has accumulated in different departments within the nursing home (social services, dietary, activities, and so forth). These documents contain valuable information describing your loved one's progress, and current and future needs.
- *Financial/insurance status.* The nursing home's financial office can provide you with an up-to-the-minute report of available Medicare benefits and secondary coverage for future in-house services, as well as an estimate of the resident's eligibility for in-home or outpatient services. If your loved one is eligible for Medicaid, the application was likely made at the time of admission, so some of the hurdles should already be cleared.

- Has the resident met the goals set by that department?
- Will the resident be able to function in the new setting?

The first question is easier than the second, and the answer is usually based on objective, numerical data gathered during the resident's stay (for example, how many feet the resident can walk, how many activities he attends each week). If the resident meets established criteria, staff will affirm that he has attained the minimum level of skill necessary for independent functioning in whatever area is being discussed at that time.

The answer to the second question is based partly on objective data, but also on the staff's "feel" for the resident. Just because a person has acquired a skill, that doesn't mean he'll use it when he needs to (motivation, discipline, and perseverence are also important). If staff are not sure of a resident's true *applied capacity* (his ability and willingness to apply his independent living skills), they'll err on the side of caution and recommend against discharge.

Family input

Families are often surprised at how much influence they have in discharge planning meetings. Their input regarding the resident's care needs is taken very seriously. Thus, a key principle for family members in discharge planning meetings: *If you have doubts, voice them now.* You might feel like a traitor for delaying discharge, but if you don't express your concerns, your loved one could be discharged prematurely, and her safety compromised. (Plus, there's no guarantee there will be a spot open in the nursing home if your loved one needs to return.)

Discharge planning meetings also provide an opportunity for families to establish exactly what they will (and will not) do for the resident after discharge. Don't be shy—the treatment team and the resident both need an honest answer here. The treatment team needs to know your anticipated level of involvement so they can forge a realistic discharge plan; the resident needs to know what you're willing to do so she can make an informed decision regarding her aftercare options. Residents often assume that family members will do whatever it takes to care for them postdischarge, but as you can imagine, that's not always true.

DECIDING WHAT YOU WILL (AND WON'T) DO
TO CARE FOR YOUR LOVED ONE

Residents are often shocked and hurt when family members refuse to resume their former caregiving roles, but things do change—especially if the resident has been in the nursing home for a while. Because this is an important decision—for you as well as your loved one—it probably warrants another family meeting to discuss your loved one's aftercare options and devise a new game plan. If you go this route, use the same strategies you used during your first family meetings.

Be forewarned: These can be difficult situations for everyone. The resident may feel abandoned; family members may feel pressured to take on burdens they can't handle. These misunderstandings can sometimes be worked through, but they can also create permanent rifts among family members. Your best bet is to make postdischarge responsibilities clear ahead of time, if possible. Failing that, you must be kind, but firm: Taking on a challenge you are not prepared to meet won't benefit anyone.

Resident input

Residents often have trouble being honest and objective in discharge planning meetings: They'll rarely say they're not ready (even if they aren't), and they'll rarely ask for more help than staff recommend (even if they'd secretly like it). Most often, residents paint an overly rosy picture of their ability to handle postdischarge responsibilities.

If your loved one is legally competent, and staff decides she can live on her own, your opposition to her discharge plans won't carry much weight. You'll have much more leverage if the physician decides that your loved one needs help in meeting her postdischarge goals. In this situation, you can refuse to take part in plans you don't agree with. You might feel guilty for doing this, but it is a powerful negotiating tool in discharge planning and important if you truly feel your loved one is not ready.

The Nuts and Bolts of Discharge: Three Key Tasks

Once nursing home staff have decided that discharge is appropriate, three issues remain: *establishing current level of care needs*, *determining the appropriate setting*, and *establishing follow-up services*. Discharge cannot proceed until all three issues have been resolved.

Establishing current level of care needs

The attending physician determines a resident's level of care needs. The physician will consider input from resident, staff, and family, but the buck stops with her. She'll decide whether the resident can live independently, and if so, how much extra help is needed. Physicians generally err on the side of caution, opting for too much care rather than too little. This is motivated by genuine concern for the patient, and by liability issues as well: The wrong determination could endanger the patient's safety and result in a lawsuit.

Determining the appropriate setting

The physician determines the resident's level of care needs, but the resident and family decide where she'll go. Nursing home staff can usually recommend follow-up service providers in the community, but since it's your decision in the end, you'll have to repeat the process you engaged in when you selected a nursing home in the first place (touring, interviewing, making financial calculations, etc.). The only difference is, you'll be looking at a different type of setting this time around—most likely assisted living or long-term care.

If your legally competent loved one insists she can handle things on her own, but the family disagrees, you may be on the receiving end of some angry accusations, threats, and guilt-trips. As before, this is where a united front can come in handy: The unified family can exert considerable pressure on the care receiver, and if she is anxious to leave the nursing home, she'll likely agree to a compromise, even if it isn't exactly what she'd hoped for. However things work out, reassure your loved one that nothing is written in stone, and that alternative arrangements will be made if the first plan doesn't go well.

Establishing follow-up services

If your loved one is transferring to an assisted living facility, things are fairly simple from the family's perspective: The new facility's admissions staff will work with the current social services staff to ensure a smooth transition.

If your loved one is returning to her home or yours, things can be a bit more complicated. In this situation, the nursing home's social services staff are responsible for ensuring that follow-up services are in place prior to discharge. They can usually provide you with a list of providers within your price range and help with paperwork and other practical details. If you prefer to hunt down your own providers, you can, but either way, you'll have to provide proof that all follow-up services ordered by the physician are in place before the resident is cleared for discharge. No proof, no discharge.

Though their legal responsibilities end when the resident leaves the facility, most nursing homes check in with former residents by phone at least once or twice, to see how follow-up services are working out. If a promised service didn't materialize, or you're unhappy with the service, let the nursing home know—they may want to stop doing business with that provider. But don't expect the nursing home to intervene on your behalf at this point: Even if they made the initial arrangement for follow-up services, you deal directly with the service providers after nursing home discharge is complete.

Legal and Financial Arrangements, Revisited

While new health care arrangements are being made, take the opportunity to update your loved one's legal and financial situations as well. The sooner you begin, the easier your task will be.

Legal (re)arrangements

When your loved one entered the nursing home, you reviewed wills and trusts, established advance directives and durable powers of attorney for health care and financial matters, and made some preliminary funeral and burial arrangements. Although the documents you put in place at that time are still legally active, the situation has changed, and these arrangements might no longer fit your needs. This is a good time to review and update these documents, but first you'll need to determine three things:

- Is your loved one satisfied?
- Are trustees and conservators comfortable with their roles?
- Do family members feel that any changes are indicated?

Your loved one probably won't have any complaints, but don't be surprised if others ask for changes. It isn't unusual for powers of attorney to decide that the responsibility was more than they'd bargained for and opt out when given the chance. Family members might also have suggestions for new legal arrangements now that the nursing home stay is over. If legal documents need to be revised, contact your attorney for advice. (Do this even if the changes seem minor to you.)

Financial (re)arrangements

If your loved one is returning to independent living, now is the time to update proxy payor agreements. People usually opt for one of three arrangements at this point:

- *The active proxy.* In some cases, your loved one might ask you to manage (or continue to manage) his finances. If you agree, your loved one will need to establish appropriate proxies in your name and joint accounts in both your names, unless these are already in place. If you go this route, it's wise to have bills, direct deposit records, and automatic payment verifications sent directly to you. It's also a good idea to establish regular "accounting" meetings, during which you and your loved one review these records. If your loved one is intimidated by financial matters, keep the reviews as simple as possible, but don't skip them altogether. Periodic updates reassure your loved one that his affairs are being managed properly—and they protect you as well, if questions ever arise about money management.

- *The "proxy-in-waiting."* Many people prefer to resume their own bill-paying and record-keeping when they leave the nursing home. However, they want to keep the current proxy arrangements in place, to simplify things in case they become incapacitated in the future. For high-functioning older adults with few cognitive or memory problems, this can be an ideal arrangement. (Remember: A proxy arrangement doesn't prevent the person from managing her own finances, it just enables another person to do it if the need arises.)

- *The proxy cancellation.* Sometimes people choose to cancel all powers of attorney, close joint accounts, and resume total responsibility for their financial affairs when they leave the nursing home. This may help the person feel more in control in the short run, but it can complicate things down the line. We don't recommend taking this route (though if you do, be sure that your loved one informs her creditors in writing of her new financial situation).

Social Security and its limitations

During his working years, it's likely that your loved one (and her employer) contributed to Social Security. Now that benefits are due, the amount your loved one will receive is determined by two things: the amount she contributed and the age at which she begins receiving benefits. Social Security benefits are determined by legally mandated formulas and adjusted periodically for inflation and other factors. The Social Security Administration can provide detailed information regarding benefit rules and regulations. (Contact them by phone at 800-772-1213 or on the Internet at www.ssa.gov.)

If your loved one's income is fixed—or increasing more slowly than inflation—careful budgeting is key. Late life is not the time to build assets by investing in volatile markets. (There's not enough time to recover your losses.) And if your loved one's living costs begin to exceed her income, she may be forced to spend her savings, shrinking her nest egg and diminishing future investment income.

The good news is, budgeting comes naturally for many older adults, particularly those raised during tough economic times. Difficulties mostly

AVOIDING FINANCIAL SCAMS

Scamming the elderly is big business. Many older folks are lonely and have access to a fair amount of money. (To the rip-off artist, your loved one's modest $15,000 nest egg looks pretty inviting.) Sadly, but understandably, many victims are too embarrassed to admit they've been scammed, and even a successful prosecution rarely results in the recovery of lost money.

If your loved one is legally competent and chooses to manage her own funds, you can't protect her from every con artist and boiler-room scammer out there. But you can help her follow some commonsense tips that apply to *all* consumers, regardless of age:

- Get information about goods or services in writing, and review the information carefully before making a decision. Don't sign anything until you're completely satisfied.
- Be especially wary of door-to-door, telephone, or Internet salespeople. "Cold calls" (offers initiated by the seller, not the buyer) are notoriously bad risks. Do not be afraid to hang up the phone or refuse to open the door: Many people have lost huge sums of money by being too polite.
- Don't give out any personal information (social security, bank account, or credit card numbers) over the telephone or Internet unless *you* initiated the contact. Even then be careful, and make sure the recipient has a legitimate need for the information.
- Be suspicious of sweepstakes, contests, free gifts, and free vacations—anything that sounds too good to be true probably is. If a gift-giver or sweepstakes representative asks for money or personal information up front (credit card numbers, social security numbers, etc.), it's a scam. Hang up.
- Don't assume people are who they say they are. Insist that service providers, law enforcement officials, and government representatives (like census workers or tax assessors) show proper identification *before* they enter your home. If you don't feel comfortable, don't let them in.

occur when your loved one relied on a now-absent spouse to manage money matters, or when your loved one's cognitive abilities are compromised by illness or other factors. It's not uncommon for an older person in this situation to make poor financial decisions, overestimating their holdings and underestimating the impact of inflation, taxes, and other "hidden" costs. This can place family members in a very awkward position, having to choose between "bailing out" their loved one or letting her suffer the consequences of poor financial planning.

THE REVERSE MORTGAGE OPTION

An increasingly popular means of supplementing retirement income is the "reverse mortgage": The homeowner receives money from a new lender, and this money need not be paid back as long as the borrower lives in the home. Some reverse mortgages are federally insured; others are private loans backed only by the solvency of the companies that sell them. Most reverse mortgages have no qualifying income restrictions, and the proceeds are generally tax-free (but the interest is not deductible until the loan is paid off). The amount of money one can borrow is based on a number of factors, including the type of loan, the borrower's age, the appraised value of the home, and current interest rates; like regular mortgages, interest rates can be fixed or variable. Money can be paid to the borrower in one lump sum, in regular monthly cash advances, as a line of credit, or as a combination of these options. The loan must be repaid when the borrower dies, sells the home, or moves.

The good news is, reverse mortgages sometimes allow "house-rich/cash-poor" seniors to age in place, rather than selling a beloved family home. But there's a downside as well. Origination fees, closing costs, and servicing fees for reverse mortgages can be very high. The borrower retains title to the property, so remains liable for all property taxes, insurance, maintenance costs, and other expenses. And at some point, the loan must be repaid, with interest, which impacts significantly the amount of money left for one's heirs.

The bottom line: Be absolutely certain that you understand the terms fully before taking a reverse mortgage, and always—*always*—consult an attorney and a Certified Financial Planner before signing any documents.

HOME MODIFICATION AND ACCESSIBILITY INFORMATION

Three organizations provide especially useful information about home modification and accessibility options:

> AbleData (sponsored by the National Institute on Disability
>   and Rehabilitation Research)
> 8630 Fenton Street
> Suite 930
> Silver Spring, MD 20910
> 800-227-0216
> www.abledata.com

> American Association of Retired Persons
> 601 E Street NW
> Washington, DC 20049
> 888-687-2277
> www.aarp.org

> ElderWeb
> 1305 Chadwick Drive
> Normal, IL 61761
> 309-451-3319
> www.elderweb.com (main page)
> www.elderweb.com/living/adapt.htm
>   (home modification page)

Making the Home Safe and Secure

As you help make your loved one legally and financially secure, don't neglect his living space. Changes may be needed here as well, to make the home safe and secure. Five principles should guide your thinking as you inspect and upgrade your loved one's home (or yours, if your loved one will be moving in with you). These are:

- keep things accessible
- minimize injury risk
- increase home security
- prepare for emergencies
- accommodate cognitive limitations

Accessibility

If your loved one was in rehab during her nursing home stay, occupational therapy staff should have made a home assessment prior to discharge. If they did, use this information: OT staff are usually good at estimating your loved one's physical skills and limitations, and the accommodations she'll need to get by on her own. Three accessibility issues are particularly important:

- *Mobility.* Many newer buildings have entry ramps, doorways and hallways wide enough for wheelchairs, bathrooms on every floor, and doors equipped with push bars or lever-style handles that can be opened easily by people with limited strength and dexterity. Older buildings usually have few of these amenities and may even have some serious structural obstacles. Sometimes these obstacles can be overcome (ramps can be built, railings and grab bars installed), but the modifications needed to make a home accessible may be be-

FEDERAL FUNDING FOR HOME MODIFICATION

Limited federal funds and low-interest loans may be available to defray home modification costs for low-income elderly, and certain accessibility-related home improvements are allowable under the current Medicaid "lookback" rules. Contact Medicaid for eligibility information. Be aware, though, that even with such help, remodelling costs can still be quite expensive—sometimes prohibitive. Consider the impact of home modification on the home's resale value and whether alternative living arrangements might make more sense from a financial standpoint.

yond your loved one's resources—and yours as well.

- *Reachability.* Making a home fully accessible means making appliances and storage areas reachable. If your loved one is wheelchair-bound, or uses a walker or cane, the freezer section of a standard "freezer on top" refrigerator may be inaccessible. (Consider purchasing a "side-by-side" model.) Overhead kitchen cabinets may be unreachable as well (ditto for medicine cabinets, closet shelves, clothes hanger bars, eye-level ovens, and prefabricated chest-high soap shelves in shower stalls). If your loved one's reach has been shortened by an illness (like arthritis) or by the need to use an assistive device (like a walker), work surfaces, counters, and tabletops may have to be lowered. The best way to tell what needs to be done is to tour the house with your loved one, taking notes on things that she can—and can't—reach easily.

- *Openability.* Accessibility doesn't end with ramps and appliances—it has to do with products and packages as well. Many prepackaged items are not easily opened by older people. (Shrink-wrapping, "childproof" bottles, and milk and juice cartons can be especially challenging.) Survey your loved one's food supplies, paper products, bath products, and medicines with an eye toward detecting and correcting openability problems. If you're not sure whether your loved one can open a product or package, have her try while you're there.

MAKING MEDICATION ACCESSIBLE

If your loved one has a complex medication schedule, be sure he knows *what* drugs must be taken, *how* they must be taken, and *when*. Consider purchasing a segmented pill container, and if necessary, set out each week's worth of pills ahead of time, with every dose in its own clearly-labelled compartment. Even if your loved one's medication needs are simple, be sure he can get to what he needs. (Replace "childproof" containers with easy-open ones.) Most important of all: If you're not 100 percent certain that your loved one can manage his own medication, make other arrangements for medication administration.

Injury prevention

Slips and falls are your main concerns here. For the older adult with a shuffling gait or balance problems, houses are dangerous places. You can't get rid of every possible hazard, but you can minimize them and make your loved one aware of them.

- *Flooring.* The floors in an old house will never be perfectly even, but you should try to secure warped floorboards as best you can. (Call in a professional if you have to.) Replace worn or torn carpeting, tack down loose edges, and remove area rugs—they slide too easily. Be sure that stair treads are firmly attached, well-marked, and easy to see. Don't use slippery waxes on wood or tile floors, and discourage your loved one from going barefoot.

HIDDEN HAZARDS IN THE HOME

Many of the greatest home hazards are those we cannot see. So check the electrical, heating, cooling, and plumbing systems, and address problems before your loved one moves in. If you have doubts about the safety of any of these systems, have a professional inspect them for you.

- *Electrical.* Make sure circuit breakers work. Test outlets for signs of shorting, and get rid of extension cord "rats' nests." Inspect appliance cords for signs of wear, and replace as needed.
- *Heating and cooling systems.* Have the furnace inspected and cleaned every year, and make sure fuel is delivered at appropriate intervals. Provide safe alternatives for temperature control and comfort if the heating or cooling systems fail (for example, electric fans, extra blankets, fire-safe space heaters).
- *Plumbing.* Check for leaks in pipes and faucets (including under-sink pipes). Install antiscald devices on shower heads and bath taps, and lower the hot water temperature a bit. Be sure that toilets flush properly. Arrange to have septic tanks pumped as needed (usually every year or two).

- *Railings.* Banisters and railings should be reinforced to support your loved one's full weight. Grab bars should be installed in showers and near toilets. Because people grab for whatever's nearby when they feel themselves losing their balance, be sure that towel bars, doorknobs, and appliance handles are as secure as possible, but remind your loved one that these fixtures really weren't designed to support adult weight—and they won't, for very long.
- *Clutter.* Most houses have an accumulation of beloved but useless decoration—fun when you're forty, dangerous when you're eighty. Smaller items that can be tripped over should be removed. For larger items, you'll need to weigh the risks and benefits of moving it. (If your loved one is so used to an item that he automatically avoids it, you might as well leave it where it is.) Install nightlights to help your loved one maneuver during late-night bathroom trips.
- *Waterworks.* Tubs are especially slippery places. In addition to grab bars and siderails, consider installing permanent non-slip strips. (Avoid suction-bottom mats—they come loose too easily.) Make sure the shower curtain doesn't funnel water onto the bathroom floor—attach weights to the bottom, if necessary. Use nonskid bathmats at tubside. (Check these frequently, and replace when the bottom becomes worn.) Areas in front of bathroom and kitchen sinks should be kept dry. (Additional nonskid bathmats may be used for this.)

Security

Three things are important here:

- *Locks, peepholes, and other barriers.* Check to see that entry doors have strong locks and peepholes your loved one can use. If the locks aren't strong enough, replace them; if the peephole's too high, lower it. Be sure your loved one has the physical strength to turn locks and keys and push back manual door bolts. Consider installing a house alarm, but be sure the resident can operate it. (Many require considerable manual dexterity and good memory as well, if a confirmation code must be entered quickly to deactivate the alarm upon entry.)

• *Sound and lighting.* Make sure that lighting—both indoor and out—is adequate. If necessary, install brighter overhead lights, or add lamps in strategic spots. If your loved one's manual dexterity is limited, consider "clap-on" or motion-sensitive switches. Telephones should have large buttons, easy-to-read numbers, and speed-dial options. If need be, install amplifiers on telephones. Consider purchasing head-phones for TV and stereo, so your loved one can listen without blasting the neighbors (especially important if your loved one lives in an apartment).

• *Landscaping.* Make sure decorative plants and bushes don't offer hiding places for intruders. (Pay particular attention to areas near windows and other other access points.) If a bush or tree represents a security risk, either trim it or get rid of it.

Emergency preparations

The three key items here are *emergency warning systems*, *emergency supplies*, and *emergency call systems*:

• *Emergency warning systems.* Be sure that smoke detectors, fire alarms, carbon mononoxide indicators, and flood alerts are in good working order. (Check the batteries at least twice a year.) Make sure your loved one can hear the alarm, or re-place it with one that will get her attention—for example, an alarm with both buzzer and flashing light. Be sure she knows what to do if the alarm goes off; if she doesn't, she might panic and hurt herself.

• *Emergency supplies.* Make sure each floor has a working fire extinguisher that is light enough for your loved one to use properly. Stock the house with battery-operated flashlights, safe alternate heat sources (nothing that involves flammable material or an open flame), and emergency water supplies.

ADDITIONAL ACCESSIBILITY TIPS

When you stock your loved one's kitchen and bath, consider the following accessibility strategies:

- Divide "economy-size" packages of food into "single serving" portions.
- Open multipack paper products (such as toilet paper or paper towels), and store them so your loved one can extract a single roll at a time, as needed.
- Commercial packaging for foods and toiletrics can be virtually unopenable if one has limited hand strength, tremors, or the use of only one hand (due to stroke, or the need to grasp a cane or walker). Experiment until you find containers that work for your loved one, and transfer foods and toiletries to these containers when restocking kitchen and bath. Plastic bottles, flip-top or pull-up caps, and wide-bottom "tip-proof" containers tend to work best.
- Consider installing wall-mounted liquid soap dispensers in showers and baths (but be sure you place them where your loved one can reach them).
- If hand strength is an issue, openers should be placed in the kitchen, bath, and other areas (so your loved one won't have to hunt around when she needs to open something).
- In most cases, the bigger the handle, the easier it is to grasp. Consider purchasing large-handled items (available through catalogs and in some stores and outlets).
- Replace manual or straight razors with "no pinch" electric models.
- Replace a manual can opener with an electric model, and heavy pots and pans with lighter ones.
- Put over-the-counter and prescription medicines on shelves that can be reached with ease.
- Consider installing an under-the-cabinet lid gripper (usually made of plastic-encased rubber), that lets a person open a jar by twisting the jar with only one hand.

Post a list of locations for all emergency supplies on the front of the refrigerator.

- *Emergency call systems.* Many areas offer emergency call systems for relatively modest prices: Your loved one gets a call button that can be worn as a necklace or bracelet, and when the button is pressed, it triggers a receiver attached to her telephone, which dials a monitoring service. Someone at the service center will then try to reach the person by phone or through a two-way intercom system. If no one answers, emergency service personnel are dispatched to the home. Some systems can be programmed to dial family or other contact people before alerting the monitoring service; others ring through to the service directly. Keep in mind that these systems are not foolproof: Batteries and phones must be in good working order, and emergency personnel must be reliable. Check with your local agency on aging to see which services they recommend.

Orienting cues and memory aids

Sometimes the biggest danger in the home is your loved one's cognitive state. An alert, oriented person can usually work through most minor household problems. A confused or flustered person cannot, and she might make things worse. You can't reverse dementia, but you can accommodate the losses to some degree. Make sure the home has orienting cues that include the current date, time, and other necessary information; place these orienting cues (clocks, calendars, schedules, reminder lists, etc.) in visible places throughout the house. You can also provide your loved one with simple instructions to follow if a problem arises, like "hit Button X on the speed-dial." Then mark the button with a bright red sticker labeled *Emergency*.

12

When It's Time to Let Go: Hospice and Beyond

The woman's skin was papery thin, pale, almost translucent. Her breathing was shallow; her eyes were closed. Every minute or so she took a deep breath, and when she did, her whole body seemed to rise and tremble with the effort. Her eyelids fluttered, and she moaned softly. She was dying.

Outside the room sat her daughter, afraid to enter. Beside the daughter sat a hospice worker. The contrast between the two women was stark: The daughter anxious, her eyes puffy red, her hand grasping a shredded tissue. Jeanette, the hospice worker—calm, relaxed, her hand resting gently on the daughter's thigh.

"What are you afraid of?" Jeanette's voice was soft, reassuring.

"I don't know," said the daughter. "It's just...I can't stand to see her like this." She licked her lips and wiped them with the tissue.

Jeanette nodded, but said nothing.

"My mother," the daughter continued, "she was always so strong. She never would have wanted me to see her this way."

"She wouldn't?"

"I don't think so."

"Are you sure?"

"I...I don't know."

Jeanette paused for a moment, and chose her words carefully. "Do you think your mother would rather be alone?"

The daughter thought. Her lips grew tight. She looked off into the distance.

"Alone!" she repeated. "No, I don't think she'd rather be alone."

The two women sat in silence. The daughter continued to look away. Her eyes were misty. Jeanette leaned in toward her, but said nothing. They stayed that way for a minute or so.

Then, without warning, a change came over the daughter. She shook her head, as if to focus her thoughts. She looked in Jeanette's eyes.

"Tell me something, would you? Honestly?"

Jeanette nodded.

"How long does she have left?"

"Not long. Maybe a few hours. A day at most."

The daughter wiped her eyes with the tissue.

"Is she in pain?"

"No."

"Are you sure?"

"Yes, I'm sure."

They sat quietly for a few moments. Then the daughter spoke.

"What should I do?"

"That's up to you."

"I should go in and be with her."

The hospice worker said nothing. The daughter looked at her, paused for a moment, and rose from her seat.

Jeanette stood as well, then, and touched the daughter's shoulder. "Shall we go in?"

"All right."

The daughter brushed the lint from her jacket and patted her hair. Jeanette held the door open, and together they entered the room.

Life has changed tremendously in the last hundred years, and so has the end of life. During our great-grandparents' generation, people usually died at home, in familiar surroundings, cared for by family members. Today, things are different: Most people die in hospitals, in unfamiliar surroundings, and the last faces we see are often those of doctors and nurses, not loved ones.

For many of us, the reality of death has become far removed from everyday life. Society protects us from the details of a loved one's death, so the event is less jarring—less disturbing—in the short term. But is this really the best approach to take? Some studies suggest that more we distance ourselves from the reality of death as it's happening, the harder it is to cope with down the line.

In this chapter we focus on the events that occur toward the end of life—the emotional reactions and physical changes that take place as death draws near, the pros and cons of aggressive end-of-life medical interventions, and the feelings that arise as we grieve the loss of a loved one.

The Pros and Cons of Aggressive Interventions

Many people opt for aggressive medical care toward the end of life, and you might find yourself faced with this decision as your loved one's health deteriorates. We can't tell you what's best for you and your loved one, but we can help you consider all sides of the issue. Here are three key questions to think about as you decide whether to begin (or continue) aggressive medical care:

- *Who is this treatment intended to benefit?* Is the intervention designed to help the patient, or is it intended to protect family members from dealing with loss?
- *How long will the benefits last?* Will the intervention extend life for weeks or months, or can it realistically be expected to extend life for a matter of hours or days?
- *How will quality of life be affected?* Is the intervention so invasive that the patient's quality of life will be severely compromised?

Arguments in favor of aggressive end-of-life care

With these questions in mind, there are valid arguments in favor of aggressive end-of-life medical interventions. These include:

- *Preservation of life.* Most of us perceive death as the enemy—an invader to be fought off as long as possible, using any means necessary. Many philosophies and religions promote the view that life is sacred, to be preserved at all costs. If you or your loved one ascribe to this view, it should certainly influence your thinking.

- *Miraculous recovery.* When someone you love is seriously ill, it is natural to pray for a last-minute "miracle," and extend life as much as possible in the hope that such a miracle will occur. Even if the likelihood of recovery is remote, many people opt for aggressive care so they feel they've done everything they can and pursued every option to its fullest.

- *Benefits to family.* If family members have been denying the reality of their loved one's death, aggressive end-of-life interventions can help them adjust to the idea. A few extra days—even a few extra hours—give people time to summon their psychological resources and deal more effectively with the situation. Aggressive interventions can create a transition period, allowing family members to move from denial to acceptance of death.

- *A chance to say good-bye.* Most people have far more "unfinished business" than they realize. Aggressive treatment provides a window of opportunity for family members to voice the belated apology or the unexpressed sentiment of love and appreciation. Aggressive treatment can also buy time for distant relatives or friends to travel to the dying person's bedside to say good-bye.

Arguments against aggressive
end-of-life care

There are also some valid arguments against aggressive end-of-life interventions. Consider these as well:

- *Increased pain and suffering.* As the body stops functioning, natural pain control mechanisms erode. Even with medication and other pain-control interventions, the process of dying can be excruciating. Extending life sometimes adds to this pain, and because some dying people lose the ability to communicate effectively, you may never know how much pain your loved one is feeling.
- *Monetary costs.* A sizeable portion of most people's total lifetime health care expenditures occur during the last few months of life. Heroic efforts aimed at keeping a failing body alive are resource- and labor-intensive, and therefore quite expensive. For those whose insurance benefits have been depleted, aggressive end-of-life care can drain family resources very quickly.
- *Diversion of resources.* Keeping a terminally ill person alive diverts medical resources from other people who might benefit more fully from the extra care. It's not easy to think about others (especially strangers) during this difficult time, but the fact remains: Dollars spent on end-of-life care are not available for other purposes.
- *Unrealistic expectations.* Fear of death and loss can make people think irrationally, leading them to forget that death is, in fact, inevitable—that it will happen no matter what anyone does. Look inside yourself, and examine your motives during this difficult time. Then ask yourself: Am I doing this to help my loved one, or to shield myself from pain?

END-OF-LIFE MEDICAL CARE:
WHEN FAMILY MEMBERS DISAGREE

When no advance directives are in place, and no one has been designated the sole durable power of attorney for health care, the result can be a no-holds-barred family battle, with all the accompanying legal, financial, and emotional costs. Families have been destroyed by such battles (hence, the value of advance directives). If this type of conflict arises, contact the local ombudsman to help mediate before things get out of hand. The service is free.

If the patient has made his wishes clear ahead of time, things are more straightforward from a legal perspective. Still, it isn't unusual for family members with different philosophies or religious beliefs to oppose the dying patient's wishes and protest loudly. There is little they can do to change your loved one's advance directives, but feuding family members can make you pretty miserable anyway, and they can put a good deal of pressure on you to see things their way.

Without clear directives to the contrary, your loved one's attending physician will do everything she can to prolong life. If the physician truly feels that nothing more can be done, she will advise you of this and defer to the family's wishes. If the family is unified, and sending a clear message, the doctor will try to accommodate their wishes (within the bounds of the law). If the family refuses to voice a preference, the doctor will do what she thinks best. If the family is sending mixed or conflicting messages, the physician tends to respond to the most forceful person—or the one who seems most litigious.

The Hospice Option

If you opt for aggressive end-of-life medical care, your loved one's physician can explain the range of interventions available, given the patient's health status and the family's financial situation. If you opt against aggressive end-of-life care, there are still many things you can do to help your loved one. The hospice option is one possibility—much more widely used now than it used to be.

What is hospice?

Hospice is a loosely knit organization of caregivers—doctors, nurses, psychologists, social workers, clergy, and others—who share a single, simple view: that death is a normal part of life. Hospice workers strive to make the dying person's final days as dignified, fulfilling, and comfortable as possible by using *palliative care* (sometimes called *comfort care*). Hospice workers devote a great deal of effort to minimizing the dying person's pain and anxiety. They also spend time with the dying person's family, providing support, respite, and information about what to expect and how to deal with it. While it can feel a bit strange to have strangers in your loved one's space at this period, it is not unusual for an intense bond between hospice worker and family member to form very quickly.

What can hospice do?

Hospice care involves three main goals: *comfort*, *pain management*, and *dignity in dying*.

- *Comfort.* Where hospice is concerned, "comfort" is what the patient says it is—nothing less, nothing more. If the patient's notion of comfort is watching cartoons on TV with a bag of potato chips, so be it. Hospice staff will try to ensure that he is not in pain and that he has access to things that make him happy. They'll attend to his basic care needs—food, water, hygiene—and work to prevent or alleviate conditions (like pressure sores) that would increase discomfort.

- *Pain management.* Oversight agencies allow physicians to prescribe larger and more frequent doses of potentially addictive drugs, like morphine, to hospice-eligible patients. While every effort is made to find pain controls that are not unduly sedating, some degree of sedation is usually considered preferable to discomfort, particularly as the end draws near. Because high doses of painkilling drugs can sometimes overload weakened organ systems, their use may actually hasten death in some patients (but legally they cannot intentionally be used for this purpose).

- *Dignity in dying.* Many people harbor fears that they will spend their last days screaming, crying, gasping for breath, and thrashing in pain. Needless to say, this is not how people want their loved ones to remember them. Hospice caregivers are skilled at managing the unpleasant symptoms of final body breakdown—incontinence, vomiting, delirium, and so forth. They've dealt with these sights, sounds, and smells before, and know how to handle them without undue fuss.

HOSPICE MYTHS AND MISPERCEPTIONS

Like so many aspects of death and dying, hospice is frequently misunderstood. Certain myths and misperceptions surround hospice care, and you, as a caregiver, should understand them.

- *Hospice is not assisted suicide.* Hospice workers do not hasten death deliberately or encourage terminally ill people to "pull the plug." Although many hospice workers oppose aggressive end-of-life medical treatments or invasive life support devices, they work with patients and their families to find care options that enhance whatever life the patient chooses.
- *Hospice is not a place.* When people think of hospice, they often picture a dark, dreary "warehouse" full of dying people. Although there are some freestanding residential hospice programs, most hospice services are offered in the patient's home or in the nursing home.
- *Hospice is not a one-way street.* We often think of hospice as the dying person's "final stop," but as we noted in Chapter 1, that's not accurate. Many people are discharged from hospice when their health improves, and Medicare allows a person to return to traditional medical care under these circumstances. If the patient's condition deteriorates, they can be declared hospice-eligible again—as many times as needed.

Who is eligible for hospice?

To become eligible for hospice, the patient's attending physician must certify that she is terminally ill—that she has six months or less to live. Because physicians hesitate to declare a person terminally ill, most people actually have less than six months left by the time they are declared hospice-eligible. If the physician's prognosis turns out to be wrong, and the patient's condition stabilizes or improves, they can be discharged from hospice and returned to other levels of care.

Who pays?

Hospice is unique—it is the only form of custodial care funded by Medicare. Once a physician declares the patient hospice-eligible, Medicare will pay for two ninety-day periods and an unlimited number of sixty-day periods in a Medicare-approved hospice program. This arrangement allows the patient to switch back and forth between hospice care and traditional medical care if his condition improves, then worsens again. (The physician must recertify the need for hospice care each time the patient's health deteriorates.)

If the patient is not Medicare-eligible, or has used up his hospice days, the family might have to pay for hospice out-of-pocket. While hospice care isn't cheap, it is much less expensive than traditional inpatient care, in part because costly rehabilitative interventions aren't being used. As with any treatment, the patient and/or his durable power of attorney for health care must consent to hospice care, and they have the right to change their minds, discontinue hospice, and resume more aggressive treatment options down the line.

Emotional Reactions to the End of Life

Regardless of whether you opt for hospice care or more aggressive interventions, the end of life brings with it a range of emotional reactions—in family members as well as the patient.

The patient's perspective

For many years, researchers thought that people went through a predictable sequence of stages as death approached: denial, anger, bargaining, depression, and acceptance. We now know that people's reactions are more

---

HOSPICE INFORMATION

You can obtain information regarding hospice philosophies and services from two national organizations:

American Academy of Hospice and Palliative Medicine
4700 West Lake Avenue
Glenview, IL 60025
847-375-4712
www.aahpm.org

Hospice Foundation of America
1621 Connecticut Avenue NW
Washington, DC 20009
800-854-3402
www.hospicefoundation.org

LIVING BENEFITS AND VIATICAL SETTLEMENTS

Once a person has been declared terminally ill, it may be possible to cash in that person's life insurance to help cover current living expenses and health care costs. Some life insurance policies permit the terminally ill person to obtain "living benefits" (also called *advanced* or *accelerated* benefits): The person can give up the policy, collect some portion of the policy's face value right now (the amounts paid vary from policy to policy), and use the money for whatever she wishes.

If your loved one's life insurance does not include a living benefits provision, you may still be able to collect a *viatical settlement* by selling the policy to a viatical settlement company, in effect making them the beneficiary of the policy. The company will typically pay the policyholder 60 to 80 percent of the face value of the policy (depending on the policyholder's life expectancy), then collect the full value of the policy when the policyholder dies. Note that viatical settlements require a great deal of paperwork (including documentation from the policyholder's physician, and a waiver from the current policy beneficiary), and it may take several months (or more) before the transaction is complete. You can obtain information regarding viatical settlements from your insurance agent.

complicated—and less predictable—than that. There are as many ways to die as there are ways to live. Some people face death philosophically, and seem at peace; others fight until the very end, resisting death in every way they can. Some dying people become preoccupied with tying up loose ends and righting past wrongs; others seem unconcerned about the past.

The bottom line: Expect the unexpected, and don't be surprised if your loved one's emotional responses run the entire gamut—from anger and panic to stoic acceptance, then back again.

The family's perspective

The prospect of a loved one's death triggers a variety of responses in family members as well—anger, sadness, fear, guilt, relief, and even joy. Oftentimes we follow our loved one's lead in responding to death: If the patient is at peace, his or her loved ones may accept death more easily. When the patient fights death, loved ones often struggle with guilt over their own very natural wishes that the whole thing be over and done. Such feelings are normal, but many people feel guilty for wishing that death would come sooner—not later—to someone they care about.

The bottom line: You, like your loved one, will likely experience a variety of conflicting emotions at this time. Don't try to fight off unpleasant or "inappropriate" feelings. You can't control your feelings that way, and besides, it's what you do—not how you feel—that counts most during your loved one's final days. (You'll have plenty of time to work through your feelings later on.)

Physical Changes at Life's End

The stages of end-of-life physical decline are influenced by many factors, including the disease process, the type of care the person is receiving, the person's pain tolerance, and his or her medication regimen. For some people, the process is slow, with subtle, gradual changes. Other people go downhill quickly, from relative health to near-death in a matter of days or even hours.

A few general principles hold true for most dying patients, and you'll likely see signs of these in your loved one.

- *Weakness and confusion: The body shuts down.* Toward the end, people become very weak. They may sleep a great deal or drift in and out of consciousness. They may not recognize familiar people or may mistake familiar people (even family members) for others, real or imagined. Dying people sometimes lose the ability to speak or understand speech; if they retain the ability to speak, what they say might not make much sense or may seem completely out of character.
- *Loss of basic bodily functions: The end draws near.* Dying people usually move very little. They may refuse food and drink, and as a result, they become dehydrated and appear shrunken or dried-up. The dying person's body temperature may rise or fall (sometimes both, at different times); they'll sweat or shiver accordingly. Their breathing may become loud and take on a rasping or gurgling sound. Unpredictable muscle contractions are common, which cause the person's limbs to twitch and jerk and their face to contort.

THE DYING PROCESS: HELPFUL AND DESTRUCTIVE CAREGIVER RESPONSES

No one can prevent a terminally ill person from dying, but if your loved one is approaching life's end, there is much you can do to help ease the process. Here are some helpful caregiver responses—and some to avoid.

HELPFUL CAREGIVER RESPONSES

- *Discussing death openly.* It's tough to do, but at some point you should bring up the subject of death, so your loved one can express her feelings. Be cautious here, and follow your loved one's lead. If she wants to talk about death, do it. If she doesn't, back off.
- *Allowing the person to share troubling things.* When people realize they're dying, they sometimes want to discuss things they've kept to themselves for a long time. While dramatic deathbed confessions aren't common, don't be surprised if you hear some things you never heard before. Let your loved one speak freely now, and work through your reactions later.
- *Acknowledging (but not sharing) your own feelings and fears.* You're probably having a lot of powerful feelings of your own at this juncture. Don't lie about them, but try not to burden your loved one either. Find someone else to comfort and console you.

DESTRUCTIVE CAREGIVER RESPONSES

- *Denying reality.* False reassurance is not helpful to dying people. It prevents them from being open about their feelings and interferes with their own grief work.
- *Putting your needs first.* Your loved one's death may be painful, but this isn't about you. As difficult as it may be, focus only on what the dying person needs right now; you'll take care of your own needs later.
- *Patronizing and minimizing.* Death is a mystery, and none of us have been there yet. You don't know how it feels to die (and even if you did, you can't know exactly how your loved one feels about it). Don't pretend to understand things you can't possibly understand. Your well-meaning efforts might be taken badly by your loved one.

MEMORIES OF LIFE AND LOSS

Certain realities of grieving, loving, loss, and mourning can't be captured by guidelines and lists—you need to learn from those who have been there. Several memoirs and works of fiction describe the emotional aspects of end-of-life care especially well, with empathy, truth, and grace:

- *Patrimony,* by Philip Roth (Simon & Schuster, 1991)
  When Philip Roth's father develops a brain tumor, those closest to Herman Roth (including his son) become intensely involved in his treatment. *Patrimony* is part tribute, part diary, but mostly a beautifully written chronicle of the ways in which a parent's health crisis can prompt those around him to re-examine their lives and their relationships.
- *Roommates,* by Max Apple (Warner Books, 1995)
  While an undergraduate at the University of Michigan, Max Apple shared an apartment with his grandfather Rocky, age 93. *Roommates* recounts the ups and downs of their somewhat conflicted relationship, including Rocky's own caregiving efforts when (at age 103) his help is needed to look after his two great-grandchildren.
- *Tuesdays with Morrie,* by Mitch Albom (Doubleday, 1997)
  Already a classic, this memoir describes a series of weekly conversations between Mitch Albom and his college mentor, a retired sociology professor from Brandeis named Morrie Schwartz. Morrie's observations on paths taken and opportunities lost offer (perhaps unintentionally) one of the most engaging discussions we've seen on how to use existential principles day by day to live a fuller life.
- *Water for Elephants,* by Sara Gruen (Algonquin Books of Chapel Hill, 2006)
  Narrated by nursing home resident Jacob Jankowski, age 90 (or 93….he's not sure), this novel recounts Jacob's early years as caregiver for animals in a traveling circus. Jacob's reflections remind us that each resident we encounter in a skilled nursing facility—no matter how poor their functioning might be right now—is a real person with a compelling story and rich life narrative.

- *The moment of death.* The moment of death is usually very subtle, so much so that family members may not realize their loved one has died. After death, the muscles relax, and the bowel and bladder empty. The person's body will begin to show the unmistakable signs of death—changes in color, stiffness, coldness—but these occur slowly and can take a long time to be noticeable.

Grieving Your Loss

Grieving the loss of a loved one takes time—it can't be rushed. In fact, trying to hurry the grieving process may actually lengthen it. Psychologists divide the grieving process (sometimes called the *grief work*) into three phases: *immediate reactions*, *short-term coping*, and *long-term survival*. Here are some common responses at each stage.

Immediate reactions

Each of us responds to death in our own way, and no single response is "better" than another. Expect to see the following reactions—alone or in combination—in those closest to the person who died.

- *Shock.* When faced with the unbearable, the mind and body may simply "shut down" for a while. This is nature's way of protecting us from too-terrible pain, numbing us temporarily so we're not overwhelmed. Shock is normal, and it's usually far more frightening to observers than to the person undergoing it (who isn't feeling much of anything).
- *Denial.* No matter how well-prepared we are intellectually, we are rarely prepared to deal with death emotionally, and the impact can be severe. Denial has a dreamlike, "this-can't-be-happening" quality to it, and people often report that they spent the first hours or days after their loved one's death in a "daze" or "haze." They may feel detached, as if watching events unfold from a distance. Like shock, denial is nature's way of shielding us during a vulnerable time: It allows us to make decisions and cope with practical matters (like funeral planning) in a neutral, detached way.
- *Breakdown.* Not everyone is blessed with a temporary cocoon of denial. Some people respond to loss with immediate, unre-

---

FUNERAL PREPARATIONS

You can obtain information regarding funeral planning (including estimated costs of various products and services) from the National Funeral Director's Association. They can be reached by phone at 800-228-6332; by mail at 13625 Bishop's Drive, Brookfield, WI 53005; or on the web at www.nfda.org.

---

strained, no-holds-barred grief. They wail, scream, beat the walls, lash out at family members and physicians, and may even try to hurt themselves. Sometimes this period of extreme upset passes by itself, but when breakdown is severe, or lasts longer than a day or two, medical or psychological interventions (such as medication or grief counseling) may be needed.

Short-term coping

We don't think of the following responses as ways of "coping," but studies show they are: Painful though these experiences may be, they help us come to grips with thoughts and feelings triggered by our loss. Take note of the short-term coping responses in those closest to the person who has died. At moderate levels, these responses help us heal, but when they become too severe, they interfere with healing and merit the attention of a physician or mental health professional.

- *Depression.* Some degree of depression is a normal reaction to loss. The depressed person may feel sad or empty, and be unable to eat, sleep, or concentrate on tasks. He or she may become preoccupied with death and dying, lose interest in usual activities, and withdraw from relationships. When depression becomes severe, the risk of suicide is very real—contact your physician without delay. (We discuss the signs of depression and suicide in Chapter 10.)
- *Anger.* Like depression, anger is a natural reaction to loss. As we think about our loved one who's now gone, we may find ourselves hating those who are still here—people less giving, less kind, "less deserving" of life. The world begins to seem like an

CHILDREN AND FUNERALS

It's natural to want to shield young ones from the reality of death, but children who don't grieve properly can develop lasting emotional scars. Rather than shielding children from death, we should help them cope with it effectively. Here's how.

- *Use straightforward, honest language.* Terms like "went to sleep" and "slipped away" can be confusing to children. It's better to use accurate terms that reflect the permanence of death (but you should also help the child understand how memories of the person will live on).
- *Encourage children to attend the funeral, but don't force them.* By age five or so, many children are capable of attending funerals, but if they don't want to, suggest an alternative (like visiting the cemetery) that will still let them be a part of the process.
- *Explain what will happen ahead of time.* If your child does want to attend the funeral, prepare them ahead of time by explaining what will happen (with special care if an open casket will be used).
- *Let them leave if they get upset.* Sometimes a child wants to attend but becomes upset during the service. If your first attempts to comfort the child are unsuccessful, or if she becomes disruptive, have her wait outside. (Appoint someone to wait with her, and work this out ahead of time.)
- *Talk to them after it's over.* Sometimes death raises questions that linger long after the funeral is done. Be prepared to talk to your child about death and dying, and if she doesn't come to you, take the initiative by asking her if she has any questions.

unjust place when we think these things, and then we react in a surprising way: Since we can't get angry at the entire world, we take it out on those closest to us (ironically, the very people trying hardest to help).

- *Guilt.* The flip side of anger is guilt. (Some psychologists think of guilt as "anger directed inward.") When we finally accept that a loved one is gone, we also realize that we've lost our opportunity to correct past mistakes. Guilt often follows and may deepen as we reflect on things we wish we'd done differently. (Some people move back and forth between anger and guilt during this stage of the grieving process.) Like depression, severe guilt brings with it the possibility of self-destructive behavior—even suicide. Be alert for troubling signs, and act on them immediately.

FUNERALS R US

As we live by the Internet, so, increasingly, do we die by the Internet. These days you can pre-plan your own funeral, order your coffin or urn, decide what type of flowers you'd like, and what sort of music should be played—all online. Internet funeral planning is an increasingly popular option among those with strong feelings about how they want their passing to be marked. The good news: It allows you to have considerable control over costs and other details. The bad news: Scammers abound. Without input from funeral professionals familiar with local laws and customs, one can easily wind up with an expensive and detailed (but illegal) plan.

Worse, some Internet funeral companies are just plain rip-off artists; others mean well but might not be financially solvent by the time their services are required. At this point in the evolution of the Internet funeral business, our advice is simple: Consider purchasing *products* (such as urns or coffins) online, but coordinate with local professionals for the actual funeral *services*. (We provide contact information for the National Funeral Director's Association at the end of the book; this organization can direct you to reputable local professionals.)

Long-term survival

Once you've acknowledged your loss, you can begin to find ways to work through it constructively. Grieving the loss of a loved one is a long, slow process—think in terms of months or years, not days or weeks. The longer and more intense your relationship with the deceased, the longer the healing process is likely to take. Don't be surprised if you're still grieving months—sometimes many months—after your loss.

You can't hurry grief, but you can do things to make the process more meaningful. These include:

• *Finding meaning in loss.* Sometimes we don't realize how impor-

THE SURVIVING SPOUSE

Sometimes forgotten in the throes of a crisis, the surviving spouse needs special care after his or her loss. Here are things to watch for, and things you can do to help.

- *Depression.* Depression can be severe after the loss of a lifelong companion. Surviving spouses (especially men) are at increased risk for suicide for up to a year following their loss—sometimes longer. If you see signs of depression or suicidal thinking in the survivor, insist he gets professional help immediately—take him to the doctor yourself, if you have to. (We discuss the signs of depression and suicide in Chapter 10.)
- *Health problems.* Studies show that surviving spouses are at increased risk for health problems: Their immune systems are depleted by the stress of grief. Don't be surprised if the survivor shows frequent bouts of illness in the months after the loss. (Don't be surprised if you do, too.) If the surviving spouse's health was fragile to begin with (due to heart disease or some other chronic medical condition), be especially vigilant for signs of deterioration.
- *Need for structure.* The surviving spouse may need extra structure now that he's on his own. You can provide this yourself, by inviting him to take part in social activities (holidays, family meals, etc.). Encourage the survivor to maintain his social contacts, rather than letting friendships lapse. Help the survivor become involved at a nearby senior center, or begin volunteer work at a local school, homeless shelter, hospital, or nursing home.

tant someone was to us until they're gone. Developing an understanding of what a loved one's life and death meant to us and others can be painful, but it helps us grieve more effectively. Solitary reflection and reminiscing will help with this process. So will intimate talks with friends and those closest to your loved one. These talks allow you to you share special memories, and free yourself of pent-up sadness, guilt, and pain.

- *Developing personal rituals.* Our cultural background and religious beliefs shape our attitudes about "proper" ways to honor someone's memory. Some people draw comfort from putting flowers on a gravesite or fulfilling formal religious obligations. For others, honoring the dead means carrying on traditions or working for causes that were important to that person—making sure her life continues to have an impact. Whatever route you choose, make a point of performing some literal, physical acts in honor of your lost loved one. Where grief work is concerned, doing is as important as thinking and feeling.

- *Creating balanced memories.* Right after a loved one dies, we tend to focus only on the good: Faults are forgotten, hurts forgiven, bad memories denied. This works in the short run, but to grieve our loss effectively, we must face up to the bad as well as the good. No one is perfect, and an important part of grief work involves accepting and acknowledging this. Until we let go of our "sanitized" memories, we can never let go of the grief. But remember: Just because someone had flaws, that doesn't mean you didn't love them—or that they didn't love you.

HOW TO KNOW WHEN GRIEVING'S DONE

There's no tried-and-true formula for knowing when your grief work is complete, but some experiences are common as grieving draws to a close. Here's what to look for:

- *Fewer mood swings.* Early in the process, you felt fragile, sensitive—the tiniest thing could set you off, with angry recriminations or helpless tears. As grief work winds down, your mood becomes more stable, your mood swings less severe.
- *More balanced memories.* As grieving begins, we idealize the lost loved one. As grief work progresses, our memories become more balanced—we can see our loved one's strengths and his limitations, too.
- *Reinvestment in life.* Part of grief work is learning to live again, in a changed world, a world without our loved one. A sure sign of this is renewed interest in life—work, sex, hobbies, friendships…whatever.
- *Feeling of closure.* It's hard to describe, but there's a feeling of closure when grieving is through. Don't watch for this, though. It will come when you least expect it—a comforting sense that you've grown and changed.
- *Joyful reminiscing.* When you can feel joy—not sorrow—as you reminisce about your loved one, you know that grieving's done. The unfinished business is as finished as it's going to get, and it's time to get on with life.

Epilogue

You've Come This Far and You've Survived

This winter was a long one—longer than any I can remember—but the first signs of spring are finally here. There's a crocus or two by the edge of the woods, some buds on the trees (not too many, but a few), and those first blades of grass poking up through the snow.

There'll be more bad days before things turn around. I realize that. Ice and wind and chilling frost—maybe even a storm or two. I'm ready for the worst, though I'm hoping for the best, and I think I'm prepared either way. I know it will warm up eventually.

It seems like forever since September, and when I look back over the months, I can see how much I've changed. I couldn't feel it while it was happening, but I sure feel it now. I'm not angry anymore, but the strange thing is, I don't know where the anger went. However it left, I'm glad it's gone.

We put up a birdhouse last week, off to the side near the maple tree. And we're putting in bulbs this year—no more waiting on that. If the squirrels get them, so what? We'll just put in some new ones when fall rolls around.

Sometimes, when I can't sleep, I lie there and wonder whether there's anything I might have done differently. I made some mistakes—that's for sure—but who doesn't? Could things have worked out better? Maybe. Can I go back and change that now? No. Still, I think about it sometimes.

Three days after we put up the birdhouse, I thought I saw something—a flash of blue. I watched through the curtains for a while, sipping my tea, but nothing came or went. I went out to take a look later that afternoon, and as I crept up close I saw twigs scattered near the base of the pole. I peeked inside, but there was no nest—just empty.

Maybe they stopped for a while and moved on. Maybe they found a better, safer place. Even if they did, I'm glad we made the offer. Sometime—maybe soon—some new ones will move in. When they do, we'll be ready.

Hopefully, your loved one's experience receiving in-home, assisted living, or nursing home care went well. But sometimes, no matter how hard we try, things just don't work out as we'd hoped. Regardless of the outcome, give yourself credit—not just for *trying*, but for *succeeding*. Succeeding means doing the best you can.

Whether your loved one's situation is resolved, or still evolving, take some time to think about all you've done. As you look back, and move forward, it will help if you…

- *Try not to dwell on regrets.* No one is perfect. Everyone makes mistakes. If you must think about these, do—but not for too long. Ponder your regrets, then move on. You can't change the past.
- *Let go of anger and guilt.* Anger and guilt are normal responses to life's changes, especially negative ones. It isn't wrong to feel angry at your loved one for disrupting your life: Let the anger come, and let it pass. It's natural, too, to feel guilty about things you might have done differently (such as spending more time with your loved one when he was healthy). Like anger, guilt won't evaporate if you ignore it. Let it come, and let it go.

- *Take care of yourself.* Change can be painful, even when it's over. Take care of yourself by managing stress, pampering yourself a bit now and then, and looking ahead to new opportunities and challenges. They won't all be easy, but you'll meet them head on and conquer them, just as you conquered this one.

- *Don't rush things.* Psychic wounds—like physical wounds— take time to heal. They can't be rushed. Expect that you'll feel bad now and then, even when a difficult situation is long past. And remember: Recovery isn't smooth, but comes in fits and starts. Don't be surprised if you take a step back every once in a while. Stop and rest, and eventually you'll move forward again.

- *Invest yourself in old things—and new ones.* Part of healing is reviving old interests and renewing old ties. As you gain energy, invest it in things you care about—people, hobbies, your job...whatever. And as time goes by, allow yourself to discover new possibilities as well—new friends, new ideas, new interests, and new causes.

- *Put it all in perspective.* No one can live a life free of challenge and change. If your loved one has had a difficult time recently, try to focus on the big picture. Think about the good times she had, the things she accomplished, the people she loved (like you), and the lives she changed. No one lives forever, but when we touch the lives of others, a part of us lives on.

- *Focus on how you've grown.* You've met a challenge and grown as a result. You wouldn't have wished for this, but it happened, and you dealt with it. You're a better person for having confronted the challenge instead of running away. You're stronger now than you were before, and more mature as well.

- *Use your new knowledge to plan for the future.* Someday you might need some extra help, just like your loved one did, or does. You've learned quite a bit about planning for the future. Think about yourself and others you love. It's never too early to use what you've learned.

LET US KNOW…

If you found some parts of this book especially useful, please let us know. If some parts of the book could be improved, let us know that, too. We wrote this book to help, and we want to learn how we can do better. So if you have a moment, please e-mail us at rfbmal@hotmail.com. We can't respond to each and every message we receive, but we will read every one carefully…you have our word on it.

Checklists, Worksheets, and Resources

Home Health Care Comparison Checklist

Provider #1: _____

Provider #2: _____

Provider #3: _____

	#1	#2	#3
Agency information			
Well-established in area:	❏	❏	❏
Known by patient's doctors:	❏	❏	❏
Works with local hospitals:	❏	❏	❏
Awards from federal or state agencies:	❏	❏	❏
Censures from federal or state agencies:	❏	❏	❏
Cost			
Total cost per day:	_____	_____	_____
Amount covered by Medicare:	_____	_____	_____

	#1	#2	#3
Amount covered by Medicaid:	____	____	____
Amount covered by other insurance	____	____	____
Total out-of-pocket costs:	____	____	____

Staffing

	#1	#2	#3
Adequate staffing patterns:	☐	☐	☐
Guaranteed coverage options:	☐	☐	☐
Specialists available, as needed:	☐	☐	☐
Emergency plans in place:	☐	☐	☐
Options for finding optimal patient-caregiver matches in place:	☐	☐	☐

Caregiver qualifications

	#1	#2	#3
All providers trained at accredited institutions:	☐	☐	☐
Professional providers certified or licensed in their specialities:	☐	☐	☐
Nonlicensed staff supervised by licensed providers:	☐	☐	☐
Caregivers experienced with patients similar to your loved one:	☐	☐	☐

References

	#1	#2	#3
Former clients generally satisfied with agency:	☐	☐	☐
Former clients generally satisfied with performance of caregivers:	☐	☐	☐
Caregivers were reliable:	☐	☐	☐
Caregivers were competent:	☐	☐	☐
Caregivers were liked by patient:	☐	☐	☐
Caregivers were liked by family:	☐	☐	☐
Problems were resolved successfully:	☐	☐	☐
Past clients would use agency again:	☐	☐	☐
Problems reported by past clients:	☐	☐	☐

Nursing Home Comparison Checklist

Facility #1: _____

Facility #2: _____

Facility #3: _____

	#1	#2	#3

Accreditation

	#1	#2	#3
Facility is Medicare certified:	❑	❑	❑
Facility accepts Medicaid:	❑	❑	❑
Facility has current state license:	❑	❑	❑
Most recent survey results are available:	❑	❑	❑
No serious violations on most recent survey:	❑	❑	❑
Facility follows posted *Resident Bill of Rights*:	❑	❑	❑

Cost

	#1	#2	#3
Costs are clearly written out:	❑	❑	❑
Total cost per month:	_____	_____	_____
Amount covered by Medicare and other insurers:	_____	_____	_____
Estimate of "extras" per month:	_____	_____	_____
Out-of-pocket costs per month:	_____	_____	_____

Services

	#1	#2	#3
Local hospitalization available:	❑	❑	❑
Facility offers physical therapy:	❑	❑	❑
Facility offers occupational therapy:	❑	❑	❑
Facility offers speech therapy:	❑	❑	❑
Facility offers other therapies:	❑	❑	❑
Facility offers social services:	❑	❑	❑

	#1	#2	#3
Laundry services available:	❐	❐	❐
Hairdressing services available:	❐	❐	❐

Medical Staff

	#1	#2	#3
Resident's doctor is on staff:	❐	❐	❐
Twenty-four-hour nursing services available:	❐	❐	❐
Direct care staff seem			
accessible/visible:	❐	❐	❐
knowledgeable:	❐	❐	❐
familiar with residents:	❐	❐	❐
competent:	❐	❐	❐
patient:	❐	❐	❐
good-humored:	❐	❐	❐
Staffing patterns are adequate:	❐	❐	❐
Staff turnover is low:	❐	❐	❐
Residents satisfied with staff:	❐	❐	❐

Location

	#1	#2	#3
Facility is in a safe neighborhood:	❐	❐	❐
Facility convenient for visitors:	❐	❐	❐
Public transportation available:	❐	❐	❐
Desired shops, services nearby:	❐	❐	❐

Physical Plant

	#1	#2	#3
Building looks clean:	❐	❐	❐
Building smells fresh:	❐	❐	❐
Facility is accessible to physically-challenged people:	❐	❐	❐
Fire and emergency plans are clearly posted around building:	❐	❐	❐
Residents' rooms seem adequate:	❐	❐	❐
Rooms have options for privacy:	❐	❐	❐

	#1	#2	#3
Temperature seems appropriate:	❏	❏	❏
Public spaces are available for visiting, special occasions:	❏	❏	❏
Linens seem clean and odor-free:	❏	❏	❏
Adequate places to walk or wheel, both indoors and outdoors:	❏	❏	❏
Facility seems "homey":	❏	❏	❏

Dietary

	#1	#2	#3
Food looks and smells appetizing:	❏	❏	❏
Meals served in pleasant environment:	❏	❏	❏
Hot foods are hot, cold foods cold:	❏	❏	❏
Portions seem adequate:	❏	❏	❏
Residents' food preferences respected:	❏	❏	❏
Alternate menus are readily available if resident doesn't want a given meal:	❏	❏	❏
Adequate staff available to help feed residents unable to feed themselves:	❏	❏	❏

Activities

	#1	#2	#3
Structured activities scheduled every day:	❏	❏	❏
Activities take place during both day and evening:	❏	❏	❏
Master schedule includes activities of interest to your loved one:	❏	❏	❏
A broad range of activities is available:	❏	❏	❏
Some off-grounds activities are routinely scheduled:	❏	❏	❏
Individual activities are scheduled for bed-fast or room-bound residents:	❏	❏	❏
Schedule provides adequate stimulation for your loved one:	❏	❏	❏

	#1	#2	#3

Milieu

	#1	#2	#3
Residents appear well-groomed and clean:	❏	❏	❏
Residents not confined to bed are dressed in street clothing during daytime hours:	❏	❏	❏
Residents interact freely:	❏	❏	❏
Residents seem content:	❏	❏	❏
Residents seem busy:	❏	❏	❏
There is some flexibility in roommate arrangements:	❏	❏	❏
Confused residents housed separately from alert and oriented residents:	❏	❏	❏
Confused or agitated residents are closely monitored by staff:	❏	❏	❏
There appear to be some residents at your loved one's level of functioning:	❏	❏	❏

Religious services

	#1	#2	#3
Residents have access to clergy of their faith:	❏	❏	❏
Residents are able to attend services of their choice:	❏	❏	❏
Residents have access to space and materials for celebrating religious observances and holidays:	❏	❏	❏

Personal Documents and Papers

It's a good idea to keep copies of this list in different places (with at least one copy stored outside the home, in case of fire). Don't forget to update the list periodically, as circumstances change.

Document   Location

Mutual fund records _____

Mortgage documents _____ _____

Deeds and titles _____

Credit card information _____

Stocks _____ _____

Bonds _____

Bank accounts:

  Checking _____ _____

  Saving _____

  CDs _____

Wills _____

Trusts _____

Living wills _____

Powers of attorney _____

Insurance documents:

  Medicare _____

  Medigap _____

  Other health _____

  Long-term care _____

  Disability _____

  Homeowner's _____

  Renter's _____

  Life _____

  Automobile _____

  Business _____

Document   Location

    Personal Umbrella _____

    Other _____

Identification cards:

    Medicare _____

    Medicaid _____

    Social security _____

    Driver's license _____

    Other _____

Retirement account documents _____

Tax records _____

Passport _____

Birth certificate _____

Adoption papers _____

Naturalization papers _____

Marriage certificate _____

Divorce decree _____

Military records _____

Cemetery deed _____

Funeral instructions/documents _____

Automobile license/title _____

Recreational vehicle license/title _____

Safe deposit box contents list _____

What to Bring to the Nursing Home

You can use this checklist as you plan your loved one's nursing home move. The list can also serve as your personal record when your loved one leaves the facility (or in case something is lost during his or her stay).

Medical equipment

Eyeglasses (including sunglasses, if needed)
Contact lenses (and lens supplies)
Hearing aids, amplifiers (with extra batteries)
Dentures or bridgework (and supplies)
Artificial limbs (including padding, etc.)
Canes, walkers, wheelchairs
Splints, braces, trusses, pessaries, supportive devices
Ostomy supplies
Medic alert bracelet or necklace

Clothing, Shoes, and Accessories

Note: Most facilities have their own checklists to itemize articles of clothing the resident brings from home. Don't forget to update your list and theirs if you bring new items after the initial move.

Daywear	Umbrella
Underwear	Belts
Nightwear	Handbags
Outerwear	Wallets
Walking shoes	Clothing protectors
Slippers	

Toiletries

Toothbrush, toothpaste,	Denture cleanser and soaking container
Dental floss, mouthwash	Denture fixative
Shampoo and conditioner	Hairspray
Soap or shower gel	Body lotion
Body powder	Antiperspirant

Toiletries (continued)

Shaving supplies
(razor, shaving cream,
aftershave lotion)
Depilatory supplies
(creams, waxes, gauze)
Manicure tools
(file, emery board,
cuticle scissors)
Incontinence products
(diapers, wipes,
barrier creams)

Tweezers
Clippers
Comb and brush
Hair dryer
Makeup
Ostomy products
(deodorant, fixative)
Feminine hygiene products
(lubricant)

Household/Entertainment

Note: You should include operating instructions for any complex equipment—don't assume your loved one knows how to use it or that staff will be able to troubleshoot on short notice.

Television set
(with remote control)
Telephone
(with preprogrammed
speed dial)
Radio
CD or cassette player
Player for books on tape
AC adaptors
Extra batteries
Calendar
Computer
Computer disks
Equipment stands
(be sure they're solid)
Craft or hobby supplies
(check with facility first)

VCR
Videotapes
Answering machine
Personal address and telephone book
Pens, pencils, markers
Notecards and stationery
CDs or cassettes (labelled clearly)
Books on tape
Headphones for audio equipment
Clock
Books
Magnifiers/visual enhancers
Software/CD-ROMs
Surge protectors and adaptors
Concentrated reading lamp
Playing cards
Board games

Records a Nursing Home May Request

Even if the nursing home doesn't ask for all this information when your loved one is admitted, it's a good idea to have the information summarized and readily available.

Contact information

Names, addresses and phone numbers for:
- People to contact in case of emergency
- Durable power of attorney for health care
- Durable power of attorney for finances
- Attending physician
- Dentist
- Podiatrist
- Mortician and/or funeral home

Legal Documents

Letters of instruction in case of death
Copies of documents establishing:
- Durable power of attorney for financial matters
- Durable power of attorney for health care
- Directive to physicians ("living will")

Insurance cards/information

- Medicare
- Medicaid
- Secondary insurers
- Long-term-care insurance
- Veteran's benefits

Medical Records

- Copy of most recent physical exam and associated labwork
- Information about allergies, adverse reactions

Medical Records (continued)

Immunization records, if available
List of current medications (prescription and over-the-counter)
Information regarding special dietary needs
Admission and discharge summaries from recent hospitalizations
Reports from specialists detailing resident's health status
Mental health records

W O R K S H E E T S

Monthly Income and Expenses Worksheet

This budgeting worksheet will help you understand your loved one's cash flow (and yours as well, if you fill out a copy for yourself). If monthly expenses exceed monthly income, some tough decisions may have to be made in order to balance the budget.

Income

Monthly salary (pretax)	_____
Alimony/child support	_____
Other compensation	_____
Interest income	_____
Dividend income	_____
Other investment income	_____
Rental or business income	_____
Social security benefits	_____
Pensions	_____
IRA/Keogh	_____
Annuities	_____
Royalties	_____
Trusts	_____
Bonds	_____
Other	_____
Total monthly income:	_____

Expenses

Mortgage or rent (primary residence)	_____
Mortgage or rent (other residences)	_____
Utilities	_____
Telephone	_____

Expenses (continued)

Cable/Satellite TV   _____

Internet   _____

Home repairs   _____

Home/property maintenance   _____

Housecleaning   _____

Laundry/dry cleaning   _____

Legal/accounting fees   _____

Food   _____

Clothing   _____

Auto/transportation   _____

Medical/dental (unreimbursed)   _____

Medication (out-of-pocket costs)   _____

Gifts   _____

Travel   _____

Education   _____

Entertainment   _____

Child care/family support   _____

Pet care (including food)   _____

Charitable contributions   _____

Debt/loan payments:

    Auto   _____

    Credit cards   _____

    Other   _____

Taxes:

    Federal   _____

    State   _____

    Local   _____

    Social security   _____

    Other   _____

Insurance:

    Medicare   _____

    Medigap   _____

    Other health   _____

Expenses

Long-term care   _____

Disability   _____

Homeowner's   _____

Renter's   _____

Life   _____

Automobile   _____

Business   _____

Personal Umbrella   _____

Other   _____

Total monthly expenses: _____

Calculating a Person's Net Worth

To calculate your loved one's net worth, subtract their total liabilities from their total assets. Don't forget to update this information periodically, as circumstances change.

Assets

Cash and equivalents	_____
Stocks	_____
Bonds	_____
Mutual funds	_____
Partnerships	_____
Loans receivable	_____
Investment real estate	_____
Retirement:	
IRAs	_____
Keoghs	_____
Annuities	_____
Deferred compensation	_____
Cash value:	
Insurance	
Home	_____
Business	_____
Autos	_____
Recreational vehicles	_____
Household items	_____
Collections	_____
Total assets:	_____

Liabilities

Mortgage on primary residence	_____
Other mortgage(s)	_____
Outstanding loans:	
Auto	_____
Personal	_____
Home equity	_____
Other	_____
Other monies owed:	
Unpaid taxes	_____
Unpaid bills	_____
Credit card debt	_____
Other	_____
Total liabilities:	_____

Medical/Health History

This will be useful when your loved one meets with his or her primary physician or with specialists.

General information

Date and place of birth _____

Blood type _____

Known allergies _____

Prescription medications_____

Over-the-counter medications _____

Location of Medicare and other health insurance cards _____

_____

_____

Location of advance directives (living will, etc.) _____

_____

_____

Family history

Siblings: Current ages, health status _____

Children: Current ages, health status _____

Significant illnesses in:

　　Parents _____

　　Children _____

　　Siblings _____

Dates of marriages, divorces, spousal deaths _____

_____

_____

Significant illnesses in former and current spouses _____

_____

_____

Contact information

Next of kin _____

Person to contact in an emergency _____

Durable power of attorney for health care _____

Primary physician _____ _____

Other health care professionals:

    Dentist _____

    Opthamologist _____

    Podiatrist _____

    Mental health _____

    Other _____

Medical conditions

Type of problem	*Name of condition/Current status*
Neurological disorders	_____
Cancers	_____
Joint diseases	_____
Skin problems	_____
Vascular and cardiac diseases	_____
Metabolic/endocrine diseases	_____
Diseases of the eye	_____
Hearing problems	_____
Pulmonary diseases	_____
Renal and urinary disorders	_____
Digestive disorders	_____
Blood disorders	_____
Mental health problems	_____
Dental problems	_____
Foot conditions	_____
Other illnesses	_____

RESOURCES

Resource and Contact Information

We've included mailing addresses, phone numbers, and Internet contact information when available (though some organizations don't supply information in all three areas.). Contact information may change when organizations relocate (which happens more often than you'd think). If the telephone number doesn't work, try going online—Internet contact information rarely changes, even when a move occurs. As a last resort use directory assistance, giving the name of the organization and its most recent street address.

Accessibility/Home Modification

AbleData provides accessibility and home modification information; Seniornet provides technology resources (including Internet "how to" instructions) for seniors.

AbleData
8630 Fenton Street, Suite 930
Silver Spring, MD 20910
800-227-0216
www.abledata.com

Seniornet
900 Lafayette Street, Suite 604
Santa Clara, CA 95050
408-615-0928
www.seniornet.com

Agencies on Aging Contact Information

Your local agency on aging should be listed in the Human Services *section of the phone book. If not, you can obtain contact information through the federal government's Administration on Aging (www.aoa.dhhs.gov); use the "Key Topics" drop-down menu to access state and area Agencies on Aging.*

National Association of Area Agencies on Aging
1730 Rhode Island Avenue NW, Suite 1200
Washington, DC 20036
202-872-0888
www.n4a.org

Caregiver Resources/Support

These organizations provide a variety of resources for caregivers and other family members.

Alliance for Children and Families
1170 West Lake Park Drive
Milwaukee, WI 53224
414-359-1040
www.alliance1.org

Children of Aging Parents
P.O. Box 167
Richboro, PA 18954
800-227-7294
www.caps4caregivers.org

Family Caregiver Alliance
180 Montgomery Street, Suite 1100
San Francisco, CA 94104
415-434-3388
www.caregiver.org

National Alliance for Caregiving
4720 Montgomery Lane, 5th Floor
Bethesda, MD 20814
301-718-8444
www.caregiving.org

Elder Abuse

If you suspect that elder abuse has taken place, you should report it immediately. You can report your concerns to the local Elder Abuse program. (Their telephone number should be listed in the Human Services *section of the phone book, near the child and spouse abuse hotlines.) You can find the telephone number of your state's Elder Abuse program through the Elderweb's Online Eldercare Sourcebook (www.elderweb.com). If you don't have Internet access, you can obtain contact information for reporting suspected abuse by calling 800-677-1116.*

Eldercare Products and Services

The National Association of Professional Geriatric Care Managers can provide referrals for Geriatric Care Managers in your area. The other resources listed here provide contact information for a wide range of eldercare products and services.

American Geriatrics Society
350 Fifth Avenue, Suite 801
New York, NY 10118
212-308-1414
www.americangeriatrics.org

Eldercare Locator
800-677-1116
www.eldercare.gov

Elderweb
1305 Chadwick Drive
Normal, IL 61761
309-451-3319
www.elderweb.com

National Association of Professional
 Geriatric Care Managers
1604 North Country Club Road
Tucson, AZ 85716
520-881-8008
www.caremanager.org

Meals on Wheels Association
 of America
203 South Union Street
Alexandria, VA 22314
703 548-5558
www.mowaa.org

Financial/Legal Resources

Compassion and Choices provides legal forms and information on laws related to living wills and other health care matters. The Pension Rights Center can provide information and legal guidance regarding pensioners' rights (particularly helpful if a dispute should arise).

American Bar Association
 Commission on Law and Aging
 for the Elderly
740 15th Steeet NW
Washington, DC 20005
202-662-1000
www.abanet.org/aging

Financial Planning Association
Offices in Denver
 and Washington DC
800-322-4237
404-845-001
www.fpanet.org

Pension Rights Center
1350 Connecticut Avenue NW, Suite 206
Washington, DC 20036
202-296-3776
www.pensionrights.org

Compassion and Choices
P.O. Box 101810
Denver, CO 80250
800-247-7421
www.compassionandchoices.org

National Academy of
Elder Law Attorneys
1604 North Country Club Road
Tucson, AZ, 85716
520-881-4005
www.naela.org

Society of Financial Service
 Professionals
17 Campus Boulevard, Suite 201
Newtown Square, PA 19073
610-526-2500
www.financialpro.org

Funeral Planning

The National Funeral Director's Association has a website, a nationwide toll-free phone number, and two regional offices, each with its own mailing address and phone number.

National Funeral Director's Association
13625 Bishop's Drive
Brookfield, WI 53005
800-228-6332
262-789-1880
www.nfda.org

Health Information

These associations provide information regarding various late-life health problems. The American Medical Association and National Health Information Center also serve as clearinghouses where you can obtain additional resources in these (or other) areas.

Alzheimer's Association
225 North Michigan Avenue
Floor 17
Chicago, IL 60601
800-272-3900
312-335-8700
www.alz.org

American Diabetes Association
1701 North Beauregard Street
Alexandria, VA 22311
800-342-2383
www.diabetes.org

American Heart Association
7272 Greenville Avenue
Dallas, TX 75231
800-242-8721
www.americanheart.org

American Medical Association
515 North State Street
Chicago, IL 60610
800-621-8335
www.ama-assn.org

American Academy of
  Ophthalmology
PO Box 7424
San Francisco, CA 94120
415-561-8500
www.aao.org

American Foundation for
  Urologic Disease
1000 Corporate Boulevard
Linthicum, MD 21090
410-689-3700
www.auafoundation.org

American Lung Association
61 Broadway, 6th Floor
New York, NY 10006
800-LUNG-USA
212-315-8700
www.lungusa.org

American Podiatric Medical
   Association
9312 Old Georgetown Road
Bethesda, MD 20814
301 501-9200
www.apma.org

National Cancer Institute
Public Inquiries Office
6116 Executive Boulevard, Room 3036A
Bethesda, MD 20892
800-4-CANCER
301-435-3848
www.cancer.gov

National Institute of Neurological
   Disorders and Stroke
Office of Communications/
      Public Liaison
PO Box 5810
Bethesda, MD 20824
www.ninds.nih.gov

National Kidney Foundation
30 East 33rd Street, Suite 1100
New York, NY 10016
800-622-9010
212-889-2201
www.kidney.org

American Parkinson's Disease
   Association
135 Parkinson Avenue
Staten Island, NY 10305
800-223-2732
718-981-8001
www.apdaparkinson.org

Arthritis Foundation
P.O. Box 7669
Atlanta, GA 30357
800-283-7800
www.arthritis.org

National Health Information
   Center
PO Box 1133
Washington, DC 20013
800-336-4797
www.health.gov/nhic

National Institute on Deafness and
Other Communication Disorders
Information Clearinghouse
31 Center Drive, MSC 2320
Bethesda, MD 20892
800-241-1044
800-241-1055 (TTY)
www.nidcd.nih.gov

National Osteoporosis Foundation
1232 22nd Street NW
Washington, DC 20037
800-231-4222
www.nof.org

Home Care Agency Contact/Accreditation Information

These resources provide local contact information, as well as accreditation information for home care agencies and providers (including problems and deficiencies).

National Association for Home Care
and Hospice
228 7th Street SE
Washington, DC 20003
202-547-7424
www.nahc.org

Visiting Nurse Associations
of America
900 19th Street NW, Suite 200
Washington, DC 20006
202-384-1420
www.vnaa.org

Hospice Resources

You can learn more about hospice philosophy and practice through these organizations, which also provide local hospice contact information.

American Academy of Hospice and
Palliative Medicine
4700 West Lake Drive
Glenview, IL 60025
847-375-4712
www.aahpm.org

Hospice Foundation of America
2001 S Street NW, Suite 300
Washington, DC 20009
800-854-3402
www.hospicefoundation.org

Housing/Assisted Living

These organizations provide regional listings of accredited housing and assisted living facilities for seniors.

American Association of Homes
and Services for the Aging
2519 Connecticut Avenue NW
Washington, DC 20008
202-783-2242
www.aahsa.org

Assisted Living Federation of
America
1650 King Street, Suite 602
Alexandria, VA 22314
703-894-1805
www.alfa.org

Long-Term-Care Ombudsman Contact Information

Contact information for the local ombudsman must—by law—be posted publicly at all nursing facilities. This information is usually included with written material on patients' rights that residents receive upon admission. You can also obtain ombudsman contact information from your local agency on aging. (Check the Human Services section of your phone book.)

Medicare, Medicaid, and Other Insurance Information

You can obtain contact information for your state Medicare office by looking in the Government Offices *section of the phone book. Medicaid information is usually listed in the* Human Services *section of the phone book. If the information is not listed, try contacting HCFA or Medicare at the numbers listed below. A. M. Best and Standard & Poor's both provide useful, up-to-date ratings of private insurance companies.*

A. M. Best Company
Ambest Road
Oldwick, NJ 08858
908-439-2200
www.ambest.com

Health Insurance Association
    of America
601 Pennsylvania Avenue NW
South Building, Suite 500
Washington, DC 20004
202-778-3200
www.hiaa.org

Social Security Administration
Office of Public Inquiries
Windsor Park Building
6401 Security Boulevard
Baltimore, MD 21235
800-772-1213
www.ssa.gov

Centers for Medicare and Medicaid
    Services
7500 Security Boulevard
Baltimore, MD 21244
410-786-1000
www.cms.hhs.gov

Medicare
800-633-4227
www.medicare.gov

Standard & Poor's Insurance
    Rating Services
55 Water Street
New York, NY 10041
212-483-1000
www.standardandpoors.com

Mental Health Information

These organizations provide information regarding mental health problems, and their membership lists include licensed providers in every region of the country.

American Psychiatric Association
1000 Wilson Boulevard, Suite 1825
Arlington, VA 22209
703-907-7300
www.psych.org

National Academy of Social Workers
750 First Street NE, Suite 700
Washington, DC 20002
202-408-8600
www.naswdc.org

American Psychological
  Association
750 First Street NE
Washington, DC 20002
800-374-2721
202-336-5500
www.apa.org

National Organizations/Advocacy Groups Related to Aging

There are several nationwide advocacy groups, as well as groups for people of different ethnic and religious backgrounds.

American Association of Retired
  Persons
601 E Street NW
Washington, DC 20049
888-687-2277
www.aarp.org

Catholic Charities USA
66 Canal Center Plaza, Suite 600
Alexandria, VA 22314
703-549-1390
www.catholiccharitiesusa.org

National Caucus and Center
  on Black Aged
1220 L Street NW, Suite 800
Washington, DC 20005
202-637-8400
www.ncba-aged.org

B'nai B'rith
2020 K Street NW, 7th Floor
Washington, DC 20006
202-857-6600
www.bnaibrith.org

National Asian Pacific Center
  on Aging
Suite 914
1511 3rd Avenue
Seattle, WA 98101
206-624-1221
www.napca.org

National Council on Aging
1901 L Street NW, 4th Floor
Washington, DC 20036
202-479-1200
www.ncoa.org

National Hispanic Council on Aging
734 15th Street NW, Suite 1050
Washington, DC 20005
202-347-9733
www.nhcoa.org

National Institute on Aging
Building 31, Room 5C27
31 Center Drive, MSC 2292
Bethesda, MD 20892
301-496-1752
www.nih.gov/nia

National Indian Council on Aging
10501 Montgomery Blvd. NE
Suite 210
Albuquerque, NM 87111
505-292-2001
www.nicoa.org

Nursing Home Contact/Accreditation Information

Joint Commission on Accreditation of Heathcare Organizations provides local contact information, and accreditation information for nursing homes and other senior living facilities.

Joint Commission on Accreditation of
    Heathcare Organizations (JCAHO)
One Renaissance Boulevard
Oakbrook Terrace, IL 60181
630-792-5000
www.jointcommission.org

Physical and Occupational Therapy

These organizations provide information regarding physical and occupation therapy and lists of licensed providers.

American Occupational Therapy
    Association
4720 Montgomery Lane
PO Box 31220
Bethesda, MD 20824
301-652-2682
www.aota.org

American Physical Therapy
    Association
1111 North Fairfax Street
Alexandria, VA 22314
703-684-2782
www.apta.org

Rehabilitation Facilities

The Commission on Accreditation of Rehabilitation Facilities (CARF) is a good resource for information on rehabilitation programs and providers worldwide, as well as a place to get up-to-date information on legal and financial issues related to rehab.

CARF International
4891 East Grant Road
Tucson, AZ 85712
520-325-1044
www.carf.org

Tax Information

The IRS website is updated frequently and provides a wealth of information regarding tax regulations for seniors and caregivers.

Internal Revenue Service
1111 Constitution Avenue NW
Washington, DC 20024
800-829-1040
www.irs.gov

Veteran's Information/Resources

The VA phone number and website both provide up-to-date information regarding veteran's health benefits.

Department of Veterans Affairs
810 Vermont Avenue NW
Washington, DC 20420
877-222-8387
www.va.gov

Index

About the Authors

Robert F. Bornstein received his Ph.D. in Clinical Psychology from the State University of New York at Buffalo in 1986, completed an internship at the Upstate Medical Center in Syracuse, NY, and is Professor of Psychology at Adelphi University. Dr. Bornstein has published more than 150 articles and book chapters on personality dynamics, diagnosis, and treatment. His research has been funded by grants from the National Institute of Mental Health and the National Science Foundation, and he received the American Psychological Association's 2005 Theodore Millon Award for Excellence in Personality Research.

Mary A. Languirand received her Ph.D. in Clinical Psychology from the State University of New York at Buffalo in 1987, and completed an internship in clinical geropsychology at the R. H. Hutchings Psychiatric Center in Syracuse, NY. Dr. Languirand is coauthor of *The Thinking Skills Workbook* (Charles C. Thomas, 1980, 1984, 2000), a treatment manual for cognitive remediation in older adults. She now practices full-time in Long Island, NY, providing clinical services to individuals and families, and consulting to multidisciplinary professional teams in skilled nursing facilities.

The authors are married and live in Westbury, NY. They are also the authors of *Healthy Dependency: Leaning on Others Without Losing Yourself* (Newmarket Press, 2003).